Written Language Disorders

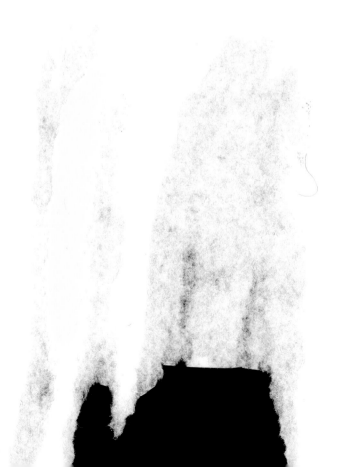

Written Language Disorders

Theory into Practice

SECOND EDITION

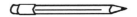

Ann M. Bain
Laura Lyons Bailet
Louisa Cook Moats

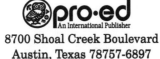
pro·ed
An International Publisher
8700 Shoal Creek Boulevard
Austin, Texas 78757-6897
800/897-3202 Fax 800/397-7633
www.proedinc.com

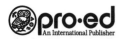

© 2001, 1991 by PRO-ED, Inc.
8700 Shoal Creek Boulevard
Austin, Texas 78757-6897
800/897-3202 Fax 800/397-7633
www.proedinc.com

Library of Congress Cataloging-in-Publication Data

Bain, Ann N.
   Written language disorders:theory into practice/Ann M. Bain. Laura Lyons Bailet,
Louisa Cook Moats.—2nd ed.
       p.   cm.
   Includes bibliographical references and index.
   ISBN 0-89079-859-1 (alk. paper)
   1. Agraphia.   2. Spelling disability.   3. Language disorders in children.   I. Bailet,
Laura Lyons.   II. Moats, Louisa Cook.   III. Title.
RC429.B34   2000
616.85'53—dc21
                                                                                        00-039962
                                                                                        CIP

This book is designed in SchoolText and New Century Schoolbook.

Printed in the United States of America

3   4   5   6   7   8   9   10   05

Contents

Chapter 6

Chapter 7

Preface

Learning to express oneself through writing is the most complex language task that children must undertake. Subsumed within written language are numerous foundation skills that are demanding in themselves. Furthermore, once an individual gains competence in these foundation skills, they must be integrated within a broader cognitive system that superimposes organizational strategies and manages issues of genre structure, text coherence and cohesion, and sense of audience. Even the most talented and prolific authors report their struggles to put words on paper in a way that best communicates their thoughts. For individuals with a specific learning disability, the most basic writing task often appears insurmountable. The purpose of this book is to review current research and theory related to written language development and disorders and to offer directions for writing instruction based upon that review. Learning to write is a protracted process. Accordingly, this book spans writing development from early childhood into the adult years.

This decade has witnessed an impressive and encouraging proliferation of research in several aspects of written language. Spelling development and disorders have received more attention than any other writing foundation skill. As Bailet and Moats point out in the first two chapters of this book, understanding of normal and deviant spelling development has broadened significantly as a result of a more comprehensive, diverse empirical database. It has become clear that learning to spell depends most critically on the emergence of advanced linguistic sensitivities, without which progress in reading and spelling typically is substantially delayed. Because of this research emphasis, approaches to assessment and treatment of spelling disorders are changing in many important ways. Gregg and Hafer present research related to written syntax, text cohesion and coherence, and text structure. Bain's chapter on handwriting reviews current theory and presents numerous methods for improving handwriting deficits.

Gould presents an overview of writing curricula, with primary emphasis on the process approach. This approach focuses on writing as a communicative attempt, rather than simply the outcome of handwriting, spelling, grammar, and punctuation combined in an additive fashion. When a process approach is used, instructional goals and methods for assessing a writing sample differ qualitatively from the more traditional product approach. Gould presents a detailed review of specific teaching methods for all stages of the writing process. In addition, she points out problems of the process approach for students with learning disabilities and suggests methods for modifying techniques and activities accordingly. In their chapter on the use of computers to foster written language development, Meyer, Murray, and Pisha also critique the product and process approaches. They present a dynamic neuropsychological framework in which to plan, execute, and evaluate remedial and developmental strategies. Computer applications in writing instruction, from prewriting to editing are reviewed in detail.

In the final chapter, Bailet reviews standardized written language tests. Although much progress has been made in terms of both the variety and psychometric characteristics of written language tests currently available, informal diagnostic assessment remains an essential component of a comprehensive evaluation. Indeed, the numerous case studies presented at the end of each chapter indicate some of the most appropriate writing activities and methods of analysis, which simply are not incorporated within current standardized writing tests.

The contributing authors of this book have their roots in teaching. Our bias, then, is to present theory and research in a scholarly manner that supports efficacious teaching methods, because only then does the theory building lead to changes that improve instruction. The chapters of this book were selected because of their potential for making that difference. For this decade we recommend that educators proceed with renewed vigor to systematically incorporate these research-based writing subskills and strategies into daily instruction. To do so will create a viable scaffolding for the foundation of written language; we understand more about the problems we seek to solve and have increasingly sophisticated curricula and technology to assist students with written language disorders in mastering the vicissitudes of writing.

Contributors

Laura Lyons Bailet, PhD
Division of Neurology
Nemours Children's Clinic
Jacksonville, FL

Ann M. Bain, EdD
Sheppard Pratt Hospital
Forbush School
Baltimore, MD

Barbara W. Gould, EdD
Department of Education
Goucher College
Baltimore, MD

Noel Gregg, PhD
Learning Disabilities Center
University of Georgia
Athens, GA

Teresa Hafer, EdS
Department of Special Education
University of Georgia
Athens, GA

Louisa Cook Moats, EdD
NICHD Early Interventions Project
Washington, DC

Anne Meyer, EdD
Center for Applied Special Technology
Peabody, MA

Elizabeth Murray, ScD
Center for Applied Special Technology
Peabody, MA

Bart Pisha, EdD
Center for Applied Special Technology
Peabody, MA

Development and Disorders of Spelling in the Beginning School Years

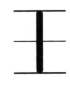

Laura Lyons Bailet

The purpose of this chapter is to review current theory, research, and educational principles related to beginning spelling development and spelling disorders in the early school years. The fundamental principle upon which this chapter is based is that spelling is predominantly a language-based activity, and spelling disability is therefore due in large part to language-based deficits. In this context, the term *language* refers not only to listening and talking, but also to an awareness of sound patterns in words and of the letters or letter sequences that we use to represent those sound patterns in print. It also refers to the ability to recognize word meaning relationships among written words by virtue of related spelling patterns. Lastly, the term *language* in this chapter includes the ability to use language to talk about words, word parts, and letter sounds. Each of these aspects of language will be described and illustrated in this chapter, as characteristics of normal spelling development and early spelling disorders are presented.

By the time normally developing children are 5 to 6 years old, they have mastered the majority of essential articulatory, syntactic, semantic, and pragmatic features of spoken language. Thus, they are able to listen, comprehend, and speak in a logical manner for conversational language and perform satisfactorily for many types of language-based learning activities. Upon enrolling in kindergarten or first grade, they face the more abstract, sophisticated linguistic tasks of learning to read and spell. These tasks involve mastery of a second-order symbol system, in that the child must associate printed symbols with their comparable spoken symbols or words (Johnson & Myklebust, 1967). They must learn that printed symbols are used in precise patterns to represent words, which in turn are symbols for objects, actions, thoughts, and feelings. In addition, they must master a new and more abstract language of instruction. Teachers begin talking about words, syllables, and letter sounds, as exemplified by the typical kindergarten task, "What is the first sound in the word *cat?*" Some children do not have the prerequisite skills necessary to comprehend this type of language, carry out the auditory analysis of letter sounds within words, or master the patterns of correspondence between letter sounds and their written counterparts. For such children, becoming competent readers and spellers may pose significant, persistent problems.

Luria (1973) described in detail the many neuropsychological processes that contribute to spelling in developing writers. According to his theory, these processes include auditory discrimination and analysis, articulation, revisualization of individual letters and letter sequences, motor programming, and motor output. For adults, it is well documented that disruption of any of these individual processes or of their integration, as occurs in brain damage, may result in markedly impaired spelling. Distinctive patterns of spelling deficits may occur in adults, depending on the location of the brain damage. Intensive study of adults, with brain damage as well as normal literate adults, has produced several theories about the specific mental processes that contribute to spelling. (For a thorough discussion, see Moats, 1995.) In children just learning to read and write, however, the cognitive organization and relative importance of these various mental processes or subskills appear to be qualitatively different from adults. A large body of empirical research has firmly established that subtle deficits in language-based phonological (auditory–linguistic) and orthographic (visual–linguistic) skills are the predominant cause of persistent reading and spelling difficulties in children (Stanovich, 1986). For this reason, the language characteristics and demands of beginning spelling will be the focus of this chapter.

Relevant Linguistic Theory

The English spelling system, or orthography, is fundamentally an alphabetic system in which phonemic units (speech sounds) are represented by graphemes (letters or letter combinations), as opposed to a writing system that represents syllables or whole words with one written symbol (Stubbs, 1980). A perfect alphabetic orthography would have only one grapheme per phoneme. English orthography clearly is not perfect in this respect, since there is more than one grapheme pattern for many phonemes. For example, the /i/ phoneme, which has the long e sound, can be spelled with graphemes ee, ea, ei, ie, e, and i. Conversely, some graphemes may have more than one pronunciation. For example, the gh grapheme combination can be pronounced as /f/ as in tough or /g/ as in ghost, or it may be silent as in though, depending upon the word in which it appears. Thus, our spelling system does not function as a simple transcription of spoken English (Smith, 1980). Rather, the spelling system visually represents English pronunciation patterns through numerous complex letter–sound correspondence rules. In addition, English orthography is governed to some extent by *morpheme* patterns, which interact with phoneme–grapheme correspondence rules to yield a highly efficient, maximally readable spelling system (N. Chomsky, 1970; Klima, 1972; Smith, 1980; Stubbs, 1980; Venezky, 1967). The term *morpheme* in this context refers to the smallest meaningful units of language and includes base words, prefixes, and suffixes. This aspect of English spelling will be elaborated upon at the end of this chapter and in the next chapter. For present purposes, the essentially alphabetic nature of English spelling will remain the focus.

Phonemes, which are the most basic distinctive units of the English language, are actually abstract categories consisting of all the concrete phonetic realizations of a given phoneme in spoken words. Nearly all utterances contain more than one phoneme, and the exact phonetic realization, or pronunciation, of that phoneme is inevitably shaped by pronunciation of phonemes that precede and follow it. For example, the precise pronunciation of /t/ varies according to its location within an utterance, as well as surrounding letters (Wagner & Torgesen, 1987). This is the principle of coarticulation, whereby individual phonemes are blended into syllable units in running speech (Liberman & Shankweiler, 1985). In representing phonemic units of speech, our alphabetic spelling system transcribes spoken English only approximately. Phonetic details that are the automatic results of coarticulation are omitted. Many spelling errors made by young children result from their lack of knowledge about these implicit rules within our spelling system. For example, beginning spellers frequently substitute *d* for *t* in the middle of words (e.g., *lidl* for *little, sdil* for *still*), because the pronunciation of *t* sounds more like *d* due to the coarticulation principle.

For both children and primary-grade teachers, this fundamental relationship between spoken and written English is the single most important issue underlying the development of literacy (Stubbs, 1980). Apprehension of this relationship, both broadly and specifically, depends upon development of linguistic sensitivities that are unnecessary for competence in oral language. The ability to analyze and manipulate language structures, particularly at the phonemic level, constitutes one critical difference between the cognitive demands of oral versus written language.

The Role of Phonological Awareness in Early Reading and Spelling

In order to comprehend and express oral language, it is unnecessary to have conscious awareness of coarticulation, or even of the existence of phonemes.

In terms of phonological analysis, the ability to discriminate syllables and words is sufficient for conversational purposes. However, many investigators have shown consistently in recent years that children must acquire more explicit linguistic awareness in order to become competent in reading and spelling. Specifically, children must become consciously aware of constituent phonemes that are blended into syllables and words. They must learn to analyze the spoken syllable, which they hear as a single "pulse of sound" (Liberman & Shankweiler, 1985, p. 9), into phonemic units, in order to master the orthographic code with which speech is represented in print.

Experiments with preschoolers, kindergartners, and first-graders have shown a consistent developmental sequence in degrees of phonological awareness as children progress in their readiness for and subsequent mastery of beginning reading and spelling. Maclean, Bryant, and Bradley (1987) conducted a 15-month longitudinal study with sixty-six 3-year-olds who were tested periodically on their ability to recite nursery rhymes and to complete several rhyming and alliteration tasks. Results demonstrated that many 3-year-olds have already acquired rudimentary phonological awareness skills. Their ability to recite nursery rhymes predicted success in rhyme detection a year or more later, even when the effects of IQ and family background were controlled. Furthermore, it was found that performance on their preschool phonological tasks predicted ability to read words at 4 years of age.

The ability to detect and produce rhyme or alliteration represents a very early level of phonological awareness. Far more difficult is the skill of counting the number of phonemes in words or manipulating individual phonemes, as is required for segmentation, blending, and deletion tasks. Liberman, Shankweiler, Fischer, and Carter (1974) found that among the 4-year-olds they tested, none could count phonemes accurately in single-syllable words, although half of them could count syllables accurately in multisyllabic words. The same general pattern occurred among the 5-year-olds. Even among subjects just completing first grade, 30% still could not count phonemes well. Similarly, in their study of 82 first-graders, Perfetti, Beck, Bell, and Hughes (1987) found that phonemic blending ability emerged early and was predictive of early reading success, whereas phoneme deletion skills (e.g., if you delete the /b/ from bat, you have the word at) emerged only after children had acquired early reading skills. Ehri's research (1989, 1994) also has suggested that some phonological skills develop in tandem with reading and spelling instruction and therefore are not necessary prerequisites for beginning to read and to spell.

Numerous other longitudinal studies, conducted in several languages, have shown that phonemic awareness is a powerful predictor of reading success (Alegria, Pignot, & Morais, 1982; Bradley & Bryant, 1983; Juel & Leavell, 1988; Lundberg, Olofsson, & Wall, 1980; Mann & Liberman, 1984; Vellutino & Scanlon, 1987). Several experimental training studies have added more solid evidence that phonological awareness plays a causal role in learning to read. (For a comprehensive review, see Wagner & Torgesen, 1987.) Bradley and Bryant (1985) included 65 children, ages 5 to 7 years, in an experimental study consisting of three different training procedures and a no-treatment control condition. All subjects had been selected on the basis of their poor performance on a sound categorization task. Results indicated that training in sound categorization, combined with spelling practice using plastic letters, was most effective in improving reading and spelling achievement. Children who received training in sound categorization alone, with no spelling practice, outperformed children who were trained in conceptual categorization and those who received no special training.

Vellutino and Scanlon (1987) carried out a large-scale training investigation that included second- and sixth-graders divided into normal and poor readers. The purpose was to assess the effects of five treatment conditions on good and poor spellers at younger and older age levels. The training conditions included the following: (a) phonemic segmentation training, (b) whole word training on nonsense syllables, and (c) a combination of segmentation and whole word training. Two control conditions were included as well. Results provided strong evidence that training in phonemic segmentation has a beneficial effect on word identification. Although the whole word method enabled children to perform well on words they had studied, they performed relatively more poorly on a transfer task that incorporated new words. The authors concluded that the ability to analyze word structure phonemically is essential for building a sizable reading vocabulary. They also found that such analysis skills are not sufficient for identifying words that do not follow phoneme–grapheme correspondence rules, an issue that will be discussed in later portions of this chapter.

Stanovich and his colleagues (Stanovich, 1986, 1988; Stanovich, Cunningham, & Cramer, 1984) have carried out numerous studies of phonological abilities in good and poor readers. Their results have shown that the relative severity of phonological deficits in true dyslexic children, as compared with poor readers, reliably distinguishes these two populations (Gough & Tunmer, 1986). Another large body of research has addressed interrelationships among phonological awareness, speech production, naming, auditory memory, and reading (e.g., Blachman, 1984; Catts, 1986; Denckla & Rudel, 1976; Felton & Wood, 1989; Katz, Shankweiler, & Liberman, 1982; Mann, Liberman, & Shankweiler, 1980). Felton and Wood (1989) conducted a series of studies with first-graders and found that children with reading disabilities performed significantly worse than children with attention-deficit disorder on phonological awareness tasks, confrontation naming, and rapid automatized naming tasks. These naming skills also have been shown to depend upon phonological skills.

Results of these and other studies implicate underlying deficits in phonological processing as the cause of numerous specific oral language and reading deficits. The degree of convergence within this extensive body of data indicates conclusively that phonological awareness is a primary causal factor in learning to read proficiently.

However, an unresolved issue concerns relationships between specific types of phonological tasks and specific aspects of learning to read. The current consensus opinion among researchers in this area is that some phonological skills develop spontaneously as a result of incidental, experiential learning and facilitate early success with reading and spelling instruction. More advanced phonological analysis ability, however, emerges as a consequence of reading and spelling instruction and in turn makes possible progress toward more advanced stages of literacy. Aspects of each skill support development of the others. This learning process is not merely additive; normally developing children add continuously to their previous knowledge about words, but they also constantly revise early concepts or strategies as they gain new knowledge and experience with language through print, both in reading and writing.

Relationships Between Learning To Read and Spell

Historically most of the research on beginning literacy has investigated factors related to learning to read, as opposed to learning to spell. In the past 3 decades, more systematic research has been undertaken to explore the nature of spelling development (Beers, 1980; Beers & Henderson, 1977; Bissex, 1980; C. Chomsky, 1979; Read, 1971, 1986; Templeton & Bear, 1992; Treiman, 1993). Whether learning to read and spell are simply two manifestations of a single underlying ability, or separable, distinct cognitive accomplishments continues to be debated. It is intuitively and theoretically plausible that reading and spelling represent separate points on a developmental language continuum, differing quantitatively in the amount of word knowledge necessary for accurate performance, but remaining qualitatively similar in the basic cognitive processes involved. The frequent observation that adults and children, both good and poor achievers, often read words they cannot spell, supports this view of the relationship between reading and spelling (Boder, 1971; Bryant & Bradley, 1980; Johnson & Myklebust, 1967). This phenomenon has been explained by the general principle that production is more difficult than reception, for both oral and written language. Production involves recall memory and more explicit, complete word knowledge than reception, which can proceed on the basis of recognition and tacit, partial word knowledge (Bryant & Bradley, 1980; L. Henderson & Chard, 1980).

The nature of the English orthographic system also contributes to differences between word recognition for reading versus spelling. A discrepancy exists between grapheme–phoneme rules for reading versus phoneme–grapheme rules for spelling. The latter are more ambiguous (Hanna, Hodges,

& Hanna, 1971; L. Henderson & Chard, 1980; Waters, Bruck, & Seidenberg, 1985). For example, the /f/ sound can be represented with four grapheme patterns: *f, ff, gh,* and *ph.* In contrast, when one sees an *f* in a word, it has only one possible pronunciation. This is true for most vowels and many consonants. Consequently, more precise orthographic memory, more explicit awareness of letter position constraints, and more awareness of the effects of word meaning principles on spelling are necessary, to spell a word rather than to read it (L. Henderson & Chard, 1980). This principle is illustrated by the misspelling of *cigar* in the writing of a fourth-grade boy who, in trying to write the phrase "close, but no cigar," wrote "close, but no sugar"! He represented the sound structure of *cigar* accurately but lacked the precise orthographic memory necessary to produce the correct spelling. When he read his own writing aloud, he recognized that he had written *sugar* instead of *cigar.* He thus showed perhaps a reliance on spelling by ear versus reading by eye for this particular word.

These factors become more important for longer words and for those words that do not follow common phoneme–grapheme correspondence patterns. The degree to which these factors influence academic instruction and learning is therefore dependent upon the types of words children are asked to read and spell. Waters et al. (1985) found that third-graders attempted to use phoneme–grapheme correspondence rules for both reading and spelling of single-syllable words, regardless of achievement levels in those subjects. Given that primary-grade spelling activities tend to focus on single-syllable, phonemically regular words, it is now clear that phonological processes are critical for learning to spell in the early school years.

Ehri (1987, 1989, 1994) has carried out extensive research in reading and spelling development and concludes that these skills are closely associated and reciprocal. She has proposed that children gradually master the phonological, orthographic, morphemic, semantic, and syntactic features of written words through experience with both reading and spelling, and that these various linguistic features of words become increasingly integrated or bonded (Moats, 1995). In a longitudinal study of white, middle-class first-graders, Uhry and Shepherd (1993) found that systematic instruction in phoneme segmentation for spelling resulted in significantly higher scores on several reading measures, as compared with more general phonics instruction. Skilled readers of all ages consistently demonstrate a continuous, automatic process of translating print to speech as they read, such that the relationships between spelling knowledge, word recognition, and speech sounds become inextricably linked and interdependent for life (Adams & Henry, 1997; Schlagal & Schlagal, 1992). Foorman and Francis (1994) carried out a study of first-grade children to look for evidence that beginning reading and spelling skills are interdependent. They found that their subjects were almost always able to read words they could spell. However, these subjects were not necessarily able to spell words that they could read, as they often misspelled words phonetically. Another interesting finding was that their subjects frequently misspelled exception words, such as *comb*, phonetically (e.g., *kome*), whereas they tended to misread them in a nonphonetic fashion (e.g., *cup* or *climb* for *comb*). Foorman and Francis suggested that their subjects were using partial letter–sound recognition and guessing to read exception words, whereas they relied more heavily on sounding them out when spelling. As children advance in their reading and spelling abilities, they may make a qualitative shift in their approach to these tasks and begin integrating spelling knowledge to enhance word recognition. It may be that children with reading and spelling disabilities do not develop this type of integrated word knowledge system, or at least develop it more slowly, which contributes to the persistence of their disabilities (Ehri, 1994; Frith, 1979).

Studies of Invented Spelling

Several years ago, Charles Read began examining the invented spellings of young children who had not yet received formal reading and spelling instruction (Read, 1971, 1986). He found striking consistency in the representational patterns children used, despite their lack of systematic instruction. Other researchers began their own investigations of invented spellings, and a clear developmental spelling sequence emerged from their efforts (Beers, 1980; Beers & Henderson, 1977; C. Chomsky, 1979; Marsh, Friedman, Welch, & Desberg, 1980; Read, 1975; Schlagal, 1989).

Rule-based representational strategies were discovered, not unlike those that have been documented during the development of oral language in the preschool years. In trying to spell, children use articulatory features of spoken language as the basis for their earliest strategies. For example, young writers characteristically write *chruk* for *truck* and *chran* for *train*, because pronunciation of /t/ in the *tr* blend is very close to the /ch/ sound. Similarly, they may substitute *g* or *j* for *dr* (e.g., *jrs* or *jes* for *dress, cilgen* for *children*). Beginning writers also omit *n*, *m*, and *l* embedded within consonant clusters, such as the *n* in *sand* or *m* in *lamp*, because they are minimally articulated. This pattern of omissions also has been observed among adult poor readers (Marcel, 1980). This articulatory strategy of representation underlies early vowel spelling patterns as well. Beginning writers tend to substitute vowels whose names are closest, in terms of articulation, to the vowel sound in question (e.g., *beg* for *big*). Another early inventive spelling strategy involves using a single letter for an entire syllable on the basis of letter names. This strategy can be seen in the spelling of *bottle* as *botl* and *candy* as *cand*.

As children gain exposure to printed language and are given systematic instruction in grapheme–phoneme and phoneme–grapheme correspondence rules, the early articulatory and letter name strategies are gradually replaced by more conventional rules. This process involves formulating, testing, and revising hypotheses about the structure of English orthography. Similar observations about the development of oral language are well documented (Berko, 1958; Derwing & Baker, 1979). For words that conform to more difficult or ambiguous orthographic patterns, or words with idiosyncratic spelling, accumulation of precise orthographic images in memory also contributes to reading and spelling proficiency (Ehri, 1980, 1989; Moats, 1995; Vellutino & Scanlon, 1987). Examples include words with vowel digraphs (e.g., *ee* and *ea*) and silent letters (e.g., ending silent *e*, or *gh* in *light*, *b* in *comb* and *climb*).

Based upon data from developmental spelling studies, children's spelling errors in the early school grades have come to be analyzed and classified according to a system that takes into account the auditory–linguistic and visual–linguistic features of English spelling, and their interaction with developing learner characteristics. These stages are described extensively in Moats (1995) and are summarized in Table 1.1.

It is emphasized that the term *stage* in this context is not meant to imply that children's spelling can be discreetly classified into one stage or another at any given time. Rather, spelling development is a continuous, protracted process with overlapping stages. Although spelling characteristics of a particular stage may predominate, there are likely to be elements of several stages present during the early school years. However, the persistence and predominance of very early, simplified spelling strategies into late second and third grades may indicate a significant spelling disability.

The journal writing samples shown in Figure 1.1 were produced by a first-grader with normally developing reading and spelling skills. Many spelling patterns characteristic of the phonetic stage can be seen. Table 1.2 shows dictated spelling responses for a 7-year, 8-month-old child in second grade who was experiencing mild to moderate difficulty with spelling in the classroom. Although he shows perhaps some transitional spelling skills (e.g., *name* and *two* spelled correctly), many of his spellings reflect the persistence of semiphonetic and early phonetic strategies. This child may have a significant disability that will require individualized instruction in order for him to advance at a reasonable pace.

Two studies have combined investigation of invented spelling with assessment of phonological abilities in kindergartners and adults who are poor spellers (Liberman, Rubin, Duques, & Carlisle, 1985; Mann, Tobin, & Wilson, 1987). Liberman and her colleagues found that, of eight language tasks administered, three accounted for 93% of the variance in invented spelling ability. These three tasks included phoneme analysis, phoneme deletion, and grapheme–phoneme matching. Similarly, Mann et al. found a significant, positive relationship between performance on a phoneme classification task and scores on an invented spelling task. In contrast, performance

Table 1.1

Stages in Spelling Development

Spelling Stage	Description	Examples
Precommunicative	Knows some letter names and recognizes some printed letters but does not understand correspondences between specific letters and sounds.	*bqx* for *man; qit* for *order*
Semiphonetic	Realizes that letters represent speech sounds. Abbreviated spellings are used, primarily consonants. Single letters often are used to represent a whole word or syllable, and beginning and ending consonants are emphasized.	*lo* for *yellow; r* for *are; u* for *you; hs* for *house; misf* for *myself*
Phonetic	Learns to represent all phonemes in a word, using knowledge of letter names and letter–sound correspondences. Spelling patterns are heavily influenced by articulatory features of phonemes and remain simplified. The *ch* sound may be represented by *h,* and the *sh* sound by *h* or *s.* The *y* sound as in *yellow* may be represented by *u,* and the *w* sound as in *water* may be represented by *y.* Long vowel sounds are represented by single letters. Short vowel sounds are represented by letters articulated in the same position.	*gen* for *green; at* for *eight; yit* for *wet; sak* for *shake; sreg* for *spring; pat* for *plant; huy* for *who; fes* for *fish; jes* for *dress; chk* or *chuk* for *truck; hk* for *chick; segeg* for *singing; haheg* for *hatching; masl* for *muscle*
Transitional	Child learns that most sounds are represented by more than one letter. Becomes aware of silent letters, double vowel patterns, double consonants, and common syllable patterns. Child may overgeneralize or undergeneralize rules and missequence letters while practicing with more advanced spelling concepts. Spellings may become less accurate phonemically during this transitional phase.	*hase* for *house; appoole* for *apple; tallist* for *tallest; cou* for *cow; lihgt* for *light; cach* for *catch; maek* for *make*

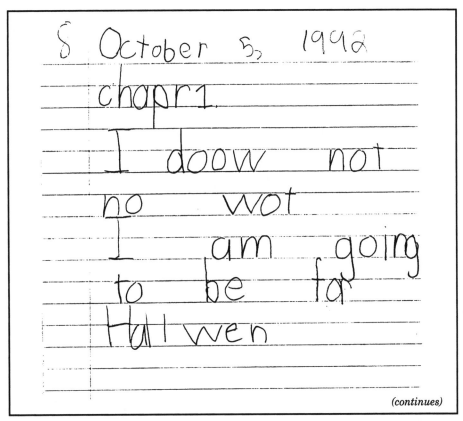

S October 5, 1992
chapr1
I doow not
no wot
I am going
to be for
Halwen

(continues)

Figure 1.1. Journal writing samples for a first-grader with normally developing spelling skills.

on a visual classification task did not correlate with scores on either the phoneme classification task or the invented spelling task.

Tangel and Blachman (1992, 1995) carried out phonemic-awareness training programs with low-income, inner-city kindergartners and first-graders and assessed the effects on invented spelling sophistication and standard spelling skills. As part of their work, they developed a reliable scoring system to evaluate the early spelling skills of kindergartners. Their results indicated developmentally superior invented spelling at the end of kindergarten for subjects receiving phonemic-awareness training, and a persistent advantage over control subjects at the end of first grade in both invented and standard spelling. The socioeconomic status of their research sample was important because other research on invented spelling generally has been conducted with children of middle- or high-income status.

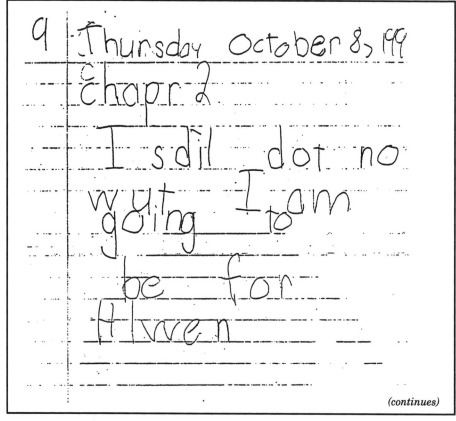

(continues)

Figure 1.1. Continued.

I recently dictated the words used in Tangel and Blachman's kindergarten study (*lap, sick, elephant, pretty, train*) to a child with a significant language disorder, for which she had attended a preschool special education classroom. She had been placed into a regular kindergarten program, but with a reduced class size of 15 students. She received 30 minutes per day of either individual or small group phonics instruction. At the end of her kindergarten year, she scored average on several individually administered reading and spelling measures and on the *Test of Phonological Awareness* (Torgesen & Bryant, 1994). Figure 1.2a shows her responses at that time for Tangel and Blachman's words, which reflect her emerging sense of sound–letter correspondences and normal spelling capabilities for her age and grade placement. Also shown is one of her spontaneous writing samples (Figure 1.2b).

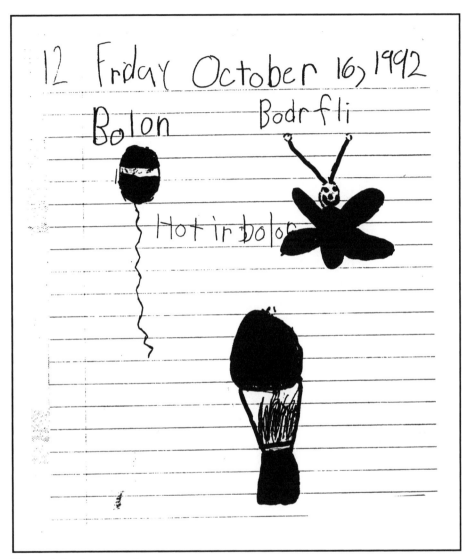

Figure 1.1. Continued.

Beginning Mastery of Morphological Spelling Principles

Whereas primary-grade children appear predominantly focused on mastering phoneme–grapheme correspondence rules for spelling, within the first 2 years of school they begin learning morphemic spelling principles as well. As mentioned earlier in this chapter, the English spelling system, although

Table 1.2
Dictation Spelling Responses of a 7-Year, 8-Month-Old Boy with Spelling Disability on the *Test of Written Spelling–Third Edition*

Dictated Word	Written Response
stop	stop
bed	bed
let	let
plant	pat
him	hem
went	yit
next	next
spring	sreg
storm	som
spend	sid
shake	sak
when	yin
yes	yes
she	sh
us	us
name	name
two	two
much	mas
myself	misf
people	pepo
who	huy
eight	at

fundamentally alphabetic, is also governed by higher level rules based on morphemic principles. These morphemic principles interact with phoneme–grapheme correspondence principles to create an efficient, readable orthography (N. Chomsky, 1970; Hodges, 1977; Klima, 1972; Smith, 1980; Stubbs, 1980; Venezky, 1967).

A simple example is the *ed* past-tense suffix, whose spelling remains the same despite three pronunciation patterns: /d/, /t/, and /əd/. The same general

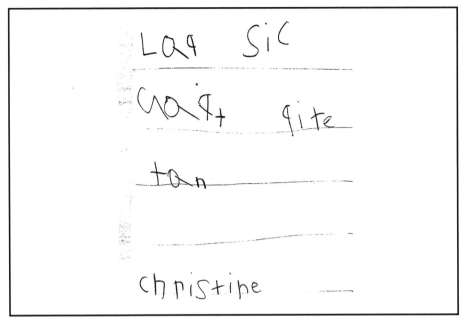

Figure 1.2a. A kindergartner's written responses for dictated words *lap, sick, elephant, pretty, train.*

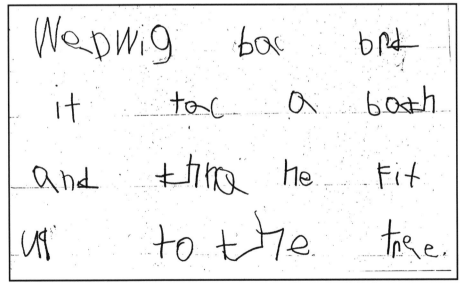

Figure 1.2b. A spontaneous writing sample for the same child during kindergarten. She read this aloud as "red wing blackbird, it take a bath and then he flew up to the tree."

principle holds true for many base word spellings that remain essentially unchanged when suffixes are added, despite pronunciation shifts. This can be seen in the case of long vowels that become schwa (unaccented) vowels when suffixes are added (e.g., *relate/relative, compete/competition*). The predictability of the phoneme–grapheme correspondence system thus is compromised to some extent, because our spelling system seeks to maintain visual similarity among words that have related meanings (Stubbs, 1980). This is true particularly for words in which pronunciation shifts are predictable and automatic. As children acquire written language, they must learn intuitively this recurring pattern of interactions and trade-offs. This process depends upon mastery of the phoneme–grapheme correspondence rule system, the higher level morphemic coding system, and integration of the two into a comprehensive, cohesive spelling system.

The work of Beers (1980) and Beers and Henderson (1977) has provided evidence of evolving morphemic knowledge in children's spelling as early as the first grade. Schwartz and Doehring (1977) also investigated young children's ability to use inflectional suffixes. They found that even beginning spellers had begun to abstract essential morphemic patterns and were able to cope with the multiple levels of linguistic representation built into the English spelling system.

Such mastery involves an ever-increasing sensitivity to various types of spelling patterns, and the ability to integrate multiple rule systems into a coherent whole. Read (1975) and Moats (1983, 1995) hypothesized that poor spelling in older students results in part from difficulty revising early spelling strategies at the normal rate to accommodate a higher level rule system. Bailet (1990) provided some empirical evidence to support this hypothesis, in a spelling study involving sixth-grade spellers with learning disabilities and younger, normally achieving spellers. Results indicated that these groups did not differ in the proportions of their spelling errors that were phonemically accurate. Thus, most subjects in both groups were able to spell reasonably well via phoneme–grapheme correspondence rules. However, the older spellers with learning disabilities wrote the *–ed* past-tense suffix significantly less accurately than the younger normally achieving spellers, who achieved nearly 100% accuracy as a group on this suffix.

Several other studies of older poor spellers' error patterns suggest that they attempt to spell using the same strategies as younger, normally achieving spellers. Nearly all of their errors can be classified within the normal developmental sequence described previously. Thus, their spelling skills tend to follow the same developmental path as normally achieving children, albeit far more slowly (Cook, 1981; Gerber, 1984; Gerber & Hall, 1987; Schwartz & Doehring, 1977). This does not mean, however, that poor spellers will become competent spellers if simply given additional time. For children with reading and spelling disabilities, significant deficits in phonological awareness, as well as other cognitive processes, prevent them from achieving as expected; therefore, they require individualized intervention. Moats's (1995) research with older poor spellers has suggested that deficits in phonological processing and the application of phoneme–grapheme correspondence rules in spelling impede the development of graphemic memory for letter sequences, even for words with less predictable or unique spellings.

Figure 1.3 shows dictated spelling responses of a 7-year, 4-month-old boy diagnosed with dyslexia. Note the primitive representational strategies he used when asked to spell plural forms for Items 19, 22, and 24. He actually drew tiny pictures of a man, a tooth, and a dress instead of trying to spell their plural forms as requested.

Assessment

The nature of any spelling assessment will depend on the purpose, the setting in which it occurs, and the training and orientation of the tester. Assessment may be undertaken to determine the progress of large groups of children, as exemplified by standardized achievement tests administered by school districts each year. Similar types of group assessments may be conducted to evaluate program effectiveness. At the level of individual child performance, assessment may be undertaken for diagnostic classification purposes, in which case the tester will rely primarily on standardized, norm-referenced instruments. The child's levels of performance relative to his or her chronological age-mates will be determined, along with score discrepancies within the child's test data, to determine whether there is evidence of a learning disability or another type of learning disorder. Several standardized spelling, handwriting, and written expression tests are reviewed in Chapter 7. Equally important is the detailed assessment of spelling error patterns across multiple writing tasks that vary in response format and degree of structure. Although responses from standardized spelling tests can provide a starting point for analyzing spelling error patterns, these tests do not provide a broad enough sample of all the major word types and patterns to derive firm conclusions. Particularly for children with limited spelling proficiency, standardized spelling tests do not provide enough items within their instructional level to ascertain emerging developmental strategies, as previously described in this chapter. The developmental spelling list and scoring system described by Tangel and Blachman (1995), described previously, is one example of functional spelling assessment for children in kindergarten and first grade. The Qualitative Inventory of Word Knowledge (E. Henderson, 1990; Schlagal, 1992) is shown and described in detail in Moats (1995) and provides instructionally relevant information on spelling in Grades 1 through 6.

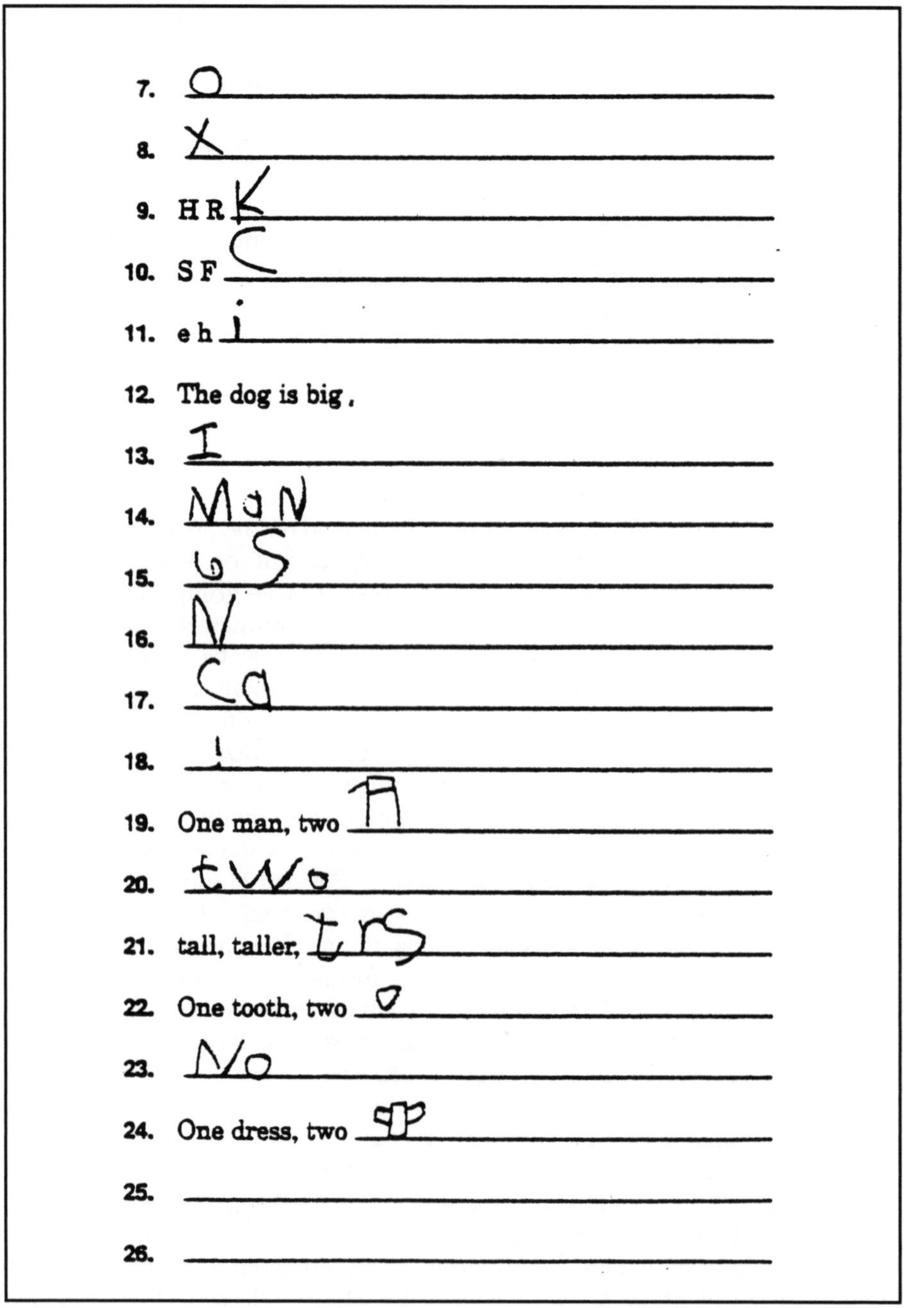

7. O

8. X

9. HR K

10. SF C

11. eh i

12. The dog is big.

13. I

14. MaN

15. 6 S

16. N

17. Ca

18. i

19. One man, two A

20. tWo

21. tall, taller, trS

22. One tooth, two ▱

23. No

24. One dress, two ▱P

25.

26.

Figure 1.3. Dictation spelling responses for a second-grade boy with dyslexia. Note the drawings as responses instead of words for Items 19, 22, and 24.

The most difficult aspect of spelling assessment is the inference of underlying process deficits based on spelling error patterns. To date, there is no universally accepted framework for this type of error analysis. Most researchers, clinicians, and test developers have tended to rely on the dichotomy of phonological versus visual or orthographic memory errors. However, as Moats (1995) pointed out, these methods often rely on superficial analysis of both word structure and learner characteristics. Familiarity and practice with error analysis based on the developmental spelling stages previously described will enable teachers to identify at least some instructional needs for individual children in the early elementary grades, and even older children with significant spelling disability. Table 1.3 and Figure 1.4 display spelling responses of a 9-year-old boy with a spelling disability. Many errors similar to those made by normally developing younger children can be seen and provide clues to the basic spelling principles and word types that need extra instruction.

Spelling disability often occurs in the context of other learning or attentional problems. For this reason, assessment of handwriting, reading, oral language, mathematics, and attentional skills should be considered along with spelling assessment. Determination of a child's global intellectual level generally is beneficial in further defining patterns of learning strengths and weaknesses and estimating probable learning rate. Given the prevalence of reading disability, which invariably is associated with spelling disability, and the causal links between poor phonological processing skills and reading disability, direct assessment of phonological analysis skills is essential in understanding the nature of the disability and developing an effective remedial plan.

Children with a history of significant oral language disorder in the preschool years are at increased risk for learning disabilities. Particularly when language comprehension problems persist, the likelihood of significant reading and spelling problems increases. Kindergarten screening for problems in phonological awareness, ability to comprehend the language of classroom instruction, and mastery of letter names and their corresponding sounds should be considered for children with a history of preschool language disorder.

Implications for Instruction

The value of encouraging young children to write without fear that their invented spellings will be marked wrong has been firmly established. Read's (1975) work on preschoolers' invented spellings highlighted the salutary effects of such an opportunity to practice writing. Simply providing children with alphabet blocks and letters, paper, and pencils encouraged early spelling attempts in children whose parents were supportive and noncritical.

Table 1.3

Spelling Responses of a 9-Year-Old Boy with Spelling Disability

Dictated Word	Written Response
go	go
cat	cat
in	een
boy	boy
and	ann
will	will
make	malk
him	hem
say	said
cut	cut
cook	cook
light	lit
must	mst
dress	jas
reach	reg
order	qit
watch	wag
enter	ent
grown	gon
nature	nagr
explain	sne

Uncorrected journal writing for several years can provide an opportunity for children to experiment with spelling patterns and expressive writing without fear of being graded down because of spelling errors. However, the need to introduce formal spelling instruction sometime during first grade is equally important, to enhance both spelling and reading progress. Exactly when and how to do this continues to be debated (Adams & Henry, 1997), but several general principles of instruction have emerged with some consensus.

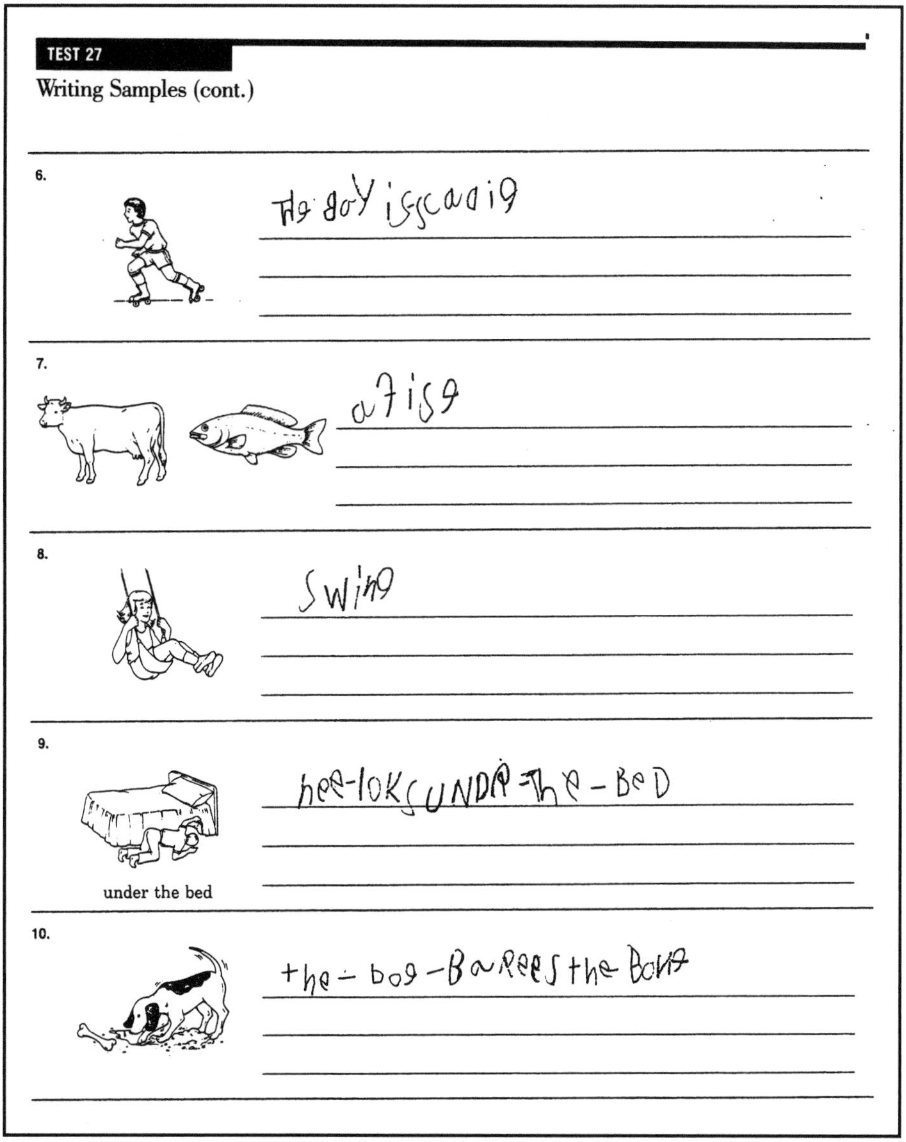

TEST 27

Writing Samples (cont.)

6.

The boy is caoi9

7.

a7is9

8.

Swi49

9.

hee-loKcUNDR-The-BeD

under the bed

10.

the-bo9-BaReeſthe Bov7

Figure 1.4. Written sentence responses for a 9-year-old boy with spelling disability.

First, the training studies cited previously, as well as many others, have demonstrated positive effects of instruction in phonological awareness on later reading and spelling performance (Bradley & Bryant, 1985; Fox & Routh, 1976, 1984; Vellutino & Scanlon, 1987). O'Connor, Notari-Syverson, and Vadasy (1996) investigated the ability of classroom teachers to incorporate phonological awareness training into their curriculum, and the impact of such instruction on phonological, reading, and writing outcomes for three groups of kindergartners: regular, repeating, and those with mild disabilities. They found that all three types of children receiving phonological awareness training performed better on outcome measures than students not receiving such training. The regular kindergarten and repeating students made more gains than the kindergartners with mild disabilities. The authors concluded that students with disabilities are likely to need more intensive, individualized instruction in phonological awareness in order to alter significantly the long-term pattern of persistent reading and spelling disabilities. Perhaps the more important result was that nearly all students benefited to some extent from phonological awareness training designed to be easily implemented in a typical classroom setting.

Phonological training procedures that provide concrete visual materials to manipulate in conjunction with auditory input appear to be most effective in improving reading and spelling achievement. Thus, for example, Bradley and Bryant (1985) gave children plastic letters to work with; Elkonin (1973) and Ball and Blachman (1991) devised similar phoneme segmentation training procedures that involve pictured objects and chips, which are placed below the picture, one chip per phoneme. These approaches to phonological awareness training share two important features that may make them beneficial to later reading and spelling achievement. First, they provide a concrete, visual means of representing spoken phonemes. Second, they provide the child with an opportunity for physically manipulating chips or letters to match their spoken counterparts, rather than requiring mental manipulation.

For example, if given a picture of *sand* and asked to identify the number of phonemes, the child can place four markers (or letters if the child is older). Suppose that the child then is shown a picture of *sad* and is asked to identify the number of phonemes. The child will place three chips or letters, thereby visually and physically experiencing the deletion of a phoneme, rather than having to carry out this process mentally. Particularly with elementary-age children and older children or adults experiencing significant reading and spelling delays, the opportunity for physical manipulation may foster phonological segmentation and blending ability. If letters are used, such procedures may also accelerate mastery of specific letter–sound correspondences. Moats (1995) provides a detailed sequence of phonological awareness tasks for both younger and older students. Most of these activities can be accomplished through short, gamelike activities that are appropriate with either individual students or groups. Snider (1995) also described in detail phonological awareness teaching techniques for use by classroom teachers.

A general teaching principle is to work from segmenting larger and more concrete units into parts, such as compound words, to segmenting smaller and more abstract units, which would include segmenting words into phonemes. The child's understanding of the task should be determined, as phonological awareness represents a completely new level of language processing that does not always spontaneously emerge as expected. I once worked with a child on segmenting compound words into parts. When I said to the child, "What would the word *sunshine* be without *sun*," the child shouted with distress, "Don't take away my sunshine!" He clearly was processing this language at a completely different level and thus did not yet demonstrate fundamental language skills to handle even a very basic phonological awareness task.

The reader is reminded that phonological awareness tasks focus primarily on specialized listening skills and thus comprise only one part of a comprehensive reading and spelling program. Simultaneously with this type of instruction, children need explicit practice in learning sound–letter and letter–sound correspondences, or phonics. Explicit phonics instruction has been proven through decades of research to result in better reading and spelling outcomes than other types of reading instruction (Foorman, 1995). Reading and spelling curricula should overlap to some extent to help children obtain adequate exposure to and practice with phonics patterns and sight vocabulary to ensure mastery. Children's attention should be focused explicitly on the pertinent spelling pattern, preferably one pattern at a time. Once a pattern is mastered, another pattern should be presented. Similarities and differences among patterns should be discussed and periodically reviewed. Instruction will be most effective if matched to the child's level of emerging skills.

Patterns of spelling responses from several writing samples should be determined, comparing error types to those associated with the various developmental spelling stages previously described. Invernizzi, Abouzeid, and Gill (1994) described a method for identifying aspects of spelling that a child has mastered, versus those for which the child has some competence, and those aspects beyond the child's developmental level. Teaching should target the middle ground. For example, if a child's spelling samples consistently indicate difficulty with short-vowel spelling patterns, instruction in long-vowel patterns is likely to be futile, as these patterns are more complex. Similarly, if a child is not yet spelling beginning and ending single consonant sounds correctly, instruction in consonant digraphs (e.g., *ch, sh, th, wh, tch, ph*) or consonant blends (e.g., *bl, br, st, mp*) would not be beneficial. The problem with standard classroom spelling instruction is that there is no individualization in the words to be learned for each weekly test. As a result, many students are asked to learn words well beyond their instructional level and miss out on an opportunity to practice at a level that would result in long-term gains. Some individualized spelling instruction within a classroom is possible, at least at a small group level, as described by Moats (1995) and Invernizzi et al. (1994).

I have long been an advocate of using word sorting activities to teach spelling patterns. Schlagal and Schlagal (1992) described a word sorting technique as a way to increase focus and flexibility in classroom spelling instruction. Consider regular, consonant–vowel–consonant (CVC) words as an example. Children can be asked to sort CVC words according to the beginning, middle, or ending letter. The teacher can identify the patterns, or the children can be asked to ascertain the patterns themselves. Word sorting activities by their nature draw attention to spelling patterns across words and enable the child to process these patterns more actively. My experience from using word sorting activities with children and adults with spelling disabilities is that the physical manipulation of word cards also facilitates learning. Many types of games can be created to extend word sorting activities.

Whereas most children require formal spelling instruction to become competent spellers, those with specific learning disabilities in reading and spelling typically require more intensive instruction over an extended time period to make long-term gains. Frequently, major deficiencies are present in phonological awareness, ability to learn letter names and sounds, and ability to identify and retain orthographic patterns. Such children often require intensive, highly structured remedial therapy, which consists of more practice than usual with each skill, and alternative techniques designed to tap the child's learning strengths while remediating learning weaknesses. For the majority of children with spelling disability, again explicit instruction in phonological awareness and phonics is essential, along with focused practice learning sight words that do not fit typical spelling patterns. *The Lindamood Phoneme Sequencing Program for Reading, Spelling, and Speech* program (Lindamood & Lindamood, 1998) is excellent for children with severe deficits in phonological awareness. Table 1.4 lists several teaching principles that can guide development of remedial programs for students with learning disabilities. Many of these principles represent simply good practices that are likely to benefit all students. Others are more specialized. The reader is again referred to Moats (1995) for additional remedial spelling strategies. In addition, many of the strategies listed are based on the work of Orton–Gillingham (Gillingham & Stillman, 1960) and Johnson and Myklebust (1967).

Finally, computers have great potential for supplementing teacher-directed activities in phonological awareness, reading, and spelling. Most children enjoy the multisensory aspect of computers and benefit from self-paced programs that provide continuous feedback. With the ever-increasing availability of home computers, families can provide opportunities for extended spelling practice at relatively low cost. The availability of spell check programs also may alleviate a child's stress about spelling errors when writing reports, and dramatically improve editing capabilities. However, it is emphasized that the computer should not be viewed as a substitute for a teacher. It is a remarkable tool that, with careful planning, can enhance a teacher's work.

Table 1.4

Remedial Teaching Strategies for Children with Spelling Difficulty

1. Avoid the tendency to work quickly in order for the child to catch up. A slow, deliberate pace will result in greater long-term gains.

2. Keep activities short, approximately 5 to 10 minutes, particularly when working with new words.

3. Limit the number of words to be learned to about three to five per day, especially if these include sight words that do not fit a pattern. More words that follow a pattern (e.g., *hop, top, mop, pop*) can be practiced in one lesson.

4. Review words daily, and introduce only one or two new words each day, depending on the child's retention.

5. Aim for at least 90% accuracy in spelling words within one pattern before introducing a new pattern. This is especially important for fundamental phonics principles, including short vowels, long vowels with ending silent *e*, single consonants, consonant blends, and consonant digraphs (*sh, ch, th, wh, tch, ph*). Many examples of each pattern should be presented, including some nonsense words that fit the pattern.

6. A synthetic or alphabetic phonics approach, which requires the child to sound out each phoneme in a word and then blend them, is an essential component of most effective remedial programs for children with learning disabilities (e.g., Gillingham & Stillman's [1960] method). For some children, particularly those with a significant articulation disorder, this may be too difficult, in which case an analytic or linguistic phonics method can be used. For these methods, the child does not sound out each phoneme, but simply says the whole word. Phonics patterns or word families still are presented systematically.

7. Use a variety of reading and spelling activities to extend practice on sight words and phonics patterns. For example, ask the child to read *–at* words (e.g., *bat, cat, fat, hat*) on cards, underline them in sentences, spell them from dictation, spell them using letter cards, write sentences with them, and play games with them.

8. Use frequent word-sorting activities.

9. For children with strong verbal skills, have them recite specific spelling rules in conjunction with word-sorting activities.

10. Experiment with multisensory techniques. Try to incorporate visual (seeing the word), auditory (hearing the word), and tactile/kinesthetic (feeling the word through touch and muscle movement) sensation. Some children learn best by seeing, saying, and tracing each letter within a word simultaneously. Others learn better by performing these steps sequentially. The child will need to study a word in this manner many times over successive days.

(continues)

Table 1.4 (Continued)

11. Present a sight word on a card (e.g., *who*) and have the child read each letter, trace it, and say the whole word. Then remove that card and present a second card on which the same word has been misspelled (e.g., *woh*). Ask the child if the word is spelled correctly. Have him or her find the error and state how to correct it. If the child has difficulty, present the original card with the correct spelling of the word for comparison. Then present a third card, with the word misspelled in a different way (e.g., *hwo*). Go through the same procedure. Continue with several cards on the same word, including some cards on which the word has been spelled correctly.

12. After several phonics patterns and sight words have been mastered, introduce the suffixes plural *–s*, past tense *–ed*, and *–ing*. Begin with words that do not require spelling changes when the suffix is added. Extended practice will be necessary to gain complete mastery of the spelling rules associated with these suffixes.

13. For words that the child has mastered, increase reading speed to encourage automaticity by using timed drills. Do not stress response speed on words the child is still learning.

14. Provide immediate corrective feedback for any errors made during a lesson.

15. Make attractive, fun charts to show children's progress and thus provide frequent positive feedback for their efforts.

Summary

This chapter has reviewed theory, research, and educational principles related to acquisition of beginning reading and spelling, as well as the problems children often encounter as they work toward becoming literate. Given that English orthography is fundamentally alphabetic, the major issue for primary students and their teachers is the abstract linguistic relationship between phonemes and graphemes.

Empirical research has established that some phonological awareness abilities are causally related to early reading and spelling achievement, and that deficits in such abilities contribute significantly to specific reading and spelling disorders. Research on children's invented spellings, as well as developmental studies of children's spelling during the first 2 years of school, has provided a broad foundation upon which current theories of spelling development and disorders are based. More research is needed to identify links between specific phonological skills, specific reading and spelling outcome measures, and their interactions with age. Nonetheless, available data support early instruction in phonological awareness, encouragement of invented spelling, and introduction of phonics-based formal spelling instruction during first grade. There is significant normal variation in the rate at which children master spelling principles and sight words. Classroom instructional methods should enable some degree of individualization of spelling lists and teaching methods. For children with persistent spelling disability, more intensive, individualized instruction is essential for an extended time period.

Case Studies

Two case studies are presented to highlight the assessment and instructional principles described in this chapter. The children's names have been changed to maintain confidentiality. In the interest of brevity and clarity, only partial test data are given.

 Jeremy

Jeremy has been seen on three occasions for psychoeducational assessment. He was initially referred during kindergarten due to poor progress in learning letter names and letter sounds. He demonstrated slow learning capabilities in essentially all academic areas, as well as significant oral language processing problems. Early language development had been delayed, in that he did not speak his first words until 2 years of age. He spoke in simple sentences at 3 years of age. After failing a speech–language screening at his school during kindergarten, he began receiving language services there. His teachers and parents had noted increasing symptoms of anxiety and fearfulness, which seemed to derive primarily from his school performance difficulties.

Some of Jeremy's psychoeducational test scores are shown in Table 1.5. There is a striking pattern of severe oral language processing problems. He displayed significant deficits in vocabulary comprehension; picture naming; short-term listening memory for sentences, words, and number strings; and verbal reasoning skills. In Jeremy's initial evaluation, phonological awareness skills were measured by the *Woodcock–Johnson–Revised Tests of Cognitive Ability* (WJ–R) (Woodcock & Johnson, 1989b), Auditory Processing cluster, and a mild deficit was noted compared with other children his age. However, his score on this cluster was higher than his scores on many other language measures. Jeremy's word pronunciation was only mildly impaired, but he displayed significant difficulty formulating grammatically correct sentences. Jeremy also displayed severe deficits in beginning academic achievement. He could write his name but could not name printed alphabet letters or write letters to dictation. Severe deficits in mathematics skills were documented as well. In

Table 1.5
Selected Psychoeducational Test Standard Scores[a] for Jeremy

| | Test Session | | |
	Test 1	Test 2	Test 3
Chronological Age	6-5	7-4	9-4
School Grade	Kindergarten	Kindergarten (repeating)	Second
Test Name			
Wechsler Intelligence Scale for Children–3			
Verbal IQ	65	NA[b]	64
Performance IQ	89	NA	96
Peabody Picture Vocabulary Test–3	66	68	85
Woodcock–Johnson–Revised Tests of Cognitive Ability			
Short-Term Memory	62	NA	83
Auditory Processing	82	NA	NA
Test of Phonological Awareness	NA	60	NA
Bender Visual Motor Gestalt Test	112	113	112
Woodcock–Johnson–Revised Tests of Achievement			
Letter–Word Identification	54	68	82
Passage Comprehension	NA	81	85
Word Attack	NA	NA	87
Calculation	NA	103	78
Applied Problems	66	75	74
Dictation	48	81	80
Writing Samples	NA	86	99
Gray Oral Reading Tests–3	NA	NA	58
Test of Written Spelling–3	NA	NA	68

[a]Standard scores have a mean of 100 and standard deviation of 15.
[b]Not administered.

contrast, Jeremy showed stronger nonverbal intellectual skills, such as working puzzles and replicating geometric patterns with blocks. His visual–motor integration skills were within the average to high average range. He was diagnosed as having a severe receptive and expressive oral language disorder and severe learning disabilities in reading, spelling, and mathematics.

Following that evaluation, Jeremy was placed into a severely language impaired, self-contained special education classroom. He repeated kindergarten in that program. Some phonics instruction took place in his classroom. He returned for a brief reassessment approximately 11 months later, at which time his mother indicated that he was progressing much better academically. She also noted that his anxiety level had decreased and that he frequently made favorable statements about his own abilities. Test scores from that evaluation are shown in Table 1.5 and indicate remarkable progress in a short period of time in reading, writing, and mathematics. He was able to name most printed alphabet letters, and he read and spelled several words. There still was evidence of severe oral language processing problems. The *Test of Phonological Awareness* (TOPA) (Torgesen & Bryant, 1994) was administered, which also indicated a severe deficit.

Jeremy remained in the same special education program through first and second grades. He returned for a third evaluation in February of second grade, at which time his anxiety level had escalated to a significant degree. His mother noted that he was unable to perform satisfactorily on his weekly spelling tests, which consisted of three- and four-syllable words (e.g., *advertise*). This was confirmed by review of his school assignments and several spelling tests. Some of the scores from the third evaluation are shown in Table 1.5. An ongoing pattern of significant language processing problems was evident, although his scores on several oral language measures had improved since his first evaluation. Persistent strengths in nonverbal skills were indicated by his increasing *Wechsler Intelligence Scale for Children–Third Edition* (WISC–III) (Wechsler, 1991) Performance IQ score and high average score on the *Bender Visual Motor Gestalt Test* (Koppitz, 1963). His scores on the *Woodcock–Johnson–Revised Tests of Achievement* (Woodcock & Johnson, 1989a) had increased in reading and written language, whereas his math scores had fallen to a mild extent. Additional reading and spelling assessment using the *Gray Oral Reading Tests–Third Edition* (Wiederholt & Bryant, 1992) and the *Test of Written Spelling–Third Edition* (TWS–3) (Larsen & Hammill, 1994) revealed persistent reading and spelling disability. Given the extent of Jeremy's learning problems, I felt that, overall, he was progressing relatively well in his cognitive, language, and academic skills. However, he remained vulnerable because of his ongoing learning deficits, and his emotional status was of major concern.

Clearly some of the instructional priorities and content had gone awry for this child, for he was not ready for the pressure of spelling three- and four-syllable words on his weekly spelling tests. He was highly motivated to succeed and became extremely stressed when persistently confronted with tasks on which failure was the likely outcome. Indeed, he had not passed a single spelling test the entire year. Immediate, complete modification of his spelling words was recommended, along with several specific teaching strategies. Table 1.6 shows his dictation spelling responses from his third evaluation,

Table 1.6
Jeremy's Spelling Responses on the *Test of Written Spelling–Third Edition*

Dictated Word	Written Response	Dictated Word	Written Response
stop	stop	yes	yes
bed	bed	she	she
let	let	us	us
plant	plat	name	name
him	hem	two	to
went	wet	much	much
next	next	myself	mysellf
spring	spring	people	pepull
storm	stom	who	hoy
spend	speed	eight	egth
shake	shack	knife	nif
when	whid	everyone	everone
hardly	hrde		

and Figure 1.5 shows his responses on a sentence writing test. Based on his pattern of spelling errors, he needed further instruction in short vowels, particularly short *e* and short *i*, and ending consonant blends for single-syllable words. Introduction of some two- and three-syllable words would be plausible, although these initially would need to follow simple CVC or VC patterns (e.g., *cabin, rabbit, velvet*). Mastery of long-vowel spelling patterns could be expected to take a long time, due to the number and complexity of patterns. Jeremy already was spelling with the inflectional suffix *–ing* (e.g., *seging* for *singing, playing* for *playing*), and some of his instruction could incorporate spelling principles related to this. He continued to need extended practice on each spelling pattern, along with work on spelling sight vocabulary (e.g., *who, what*). It was emphasized to his mother that these are the types of words and spelling patterns that are typical in second grade. His strengths needed to be emphasized, including strong sentence writing capability, as shown in Figure 1.5. Use of a computer for writing activities was recommended as a way of encouraging further writing development and creativity while minimizing the adverse impact of his spelling deficit. His mother also was encouraged to seek counseling and psychiatric consultation for Jeremy if curriculum modifications did not result in a significant reduction of his anxiety state.

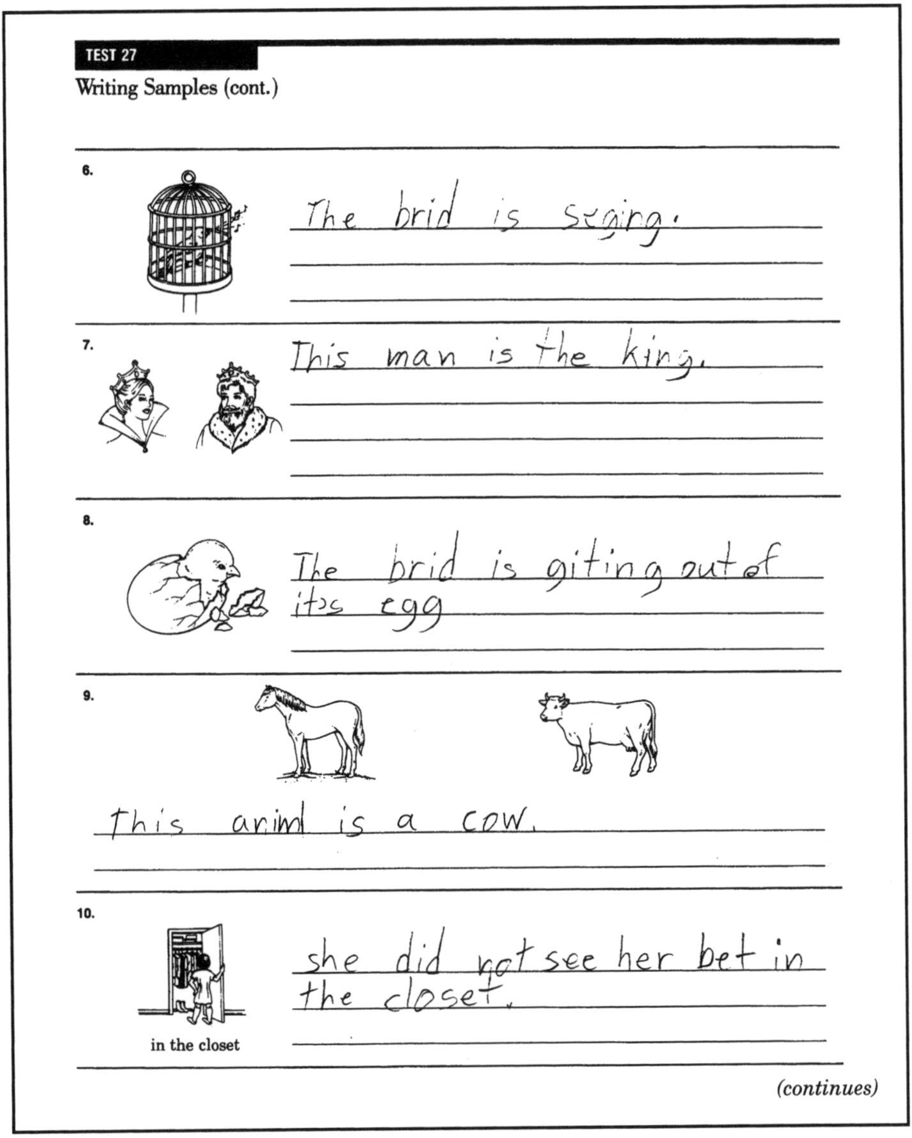

TEST 27

Writing Samples (cont.)

6. The brid is seging.

7. This man is the king.

8. The brid is giting out of its egg

9. this animl is a cow.

10.
in the closet

she did not see her bet in the closet.

(continues)

Figure 1.5. Written sentence responses for Jeremy during second grade.

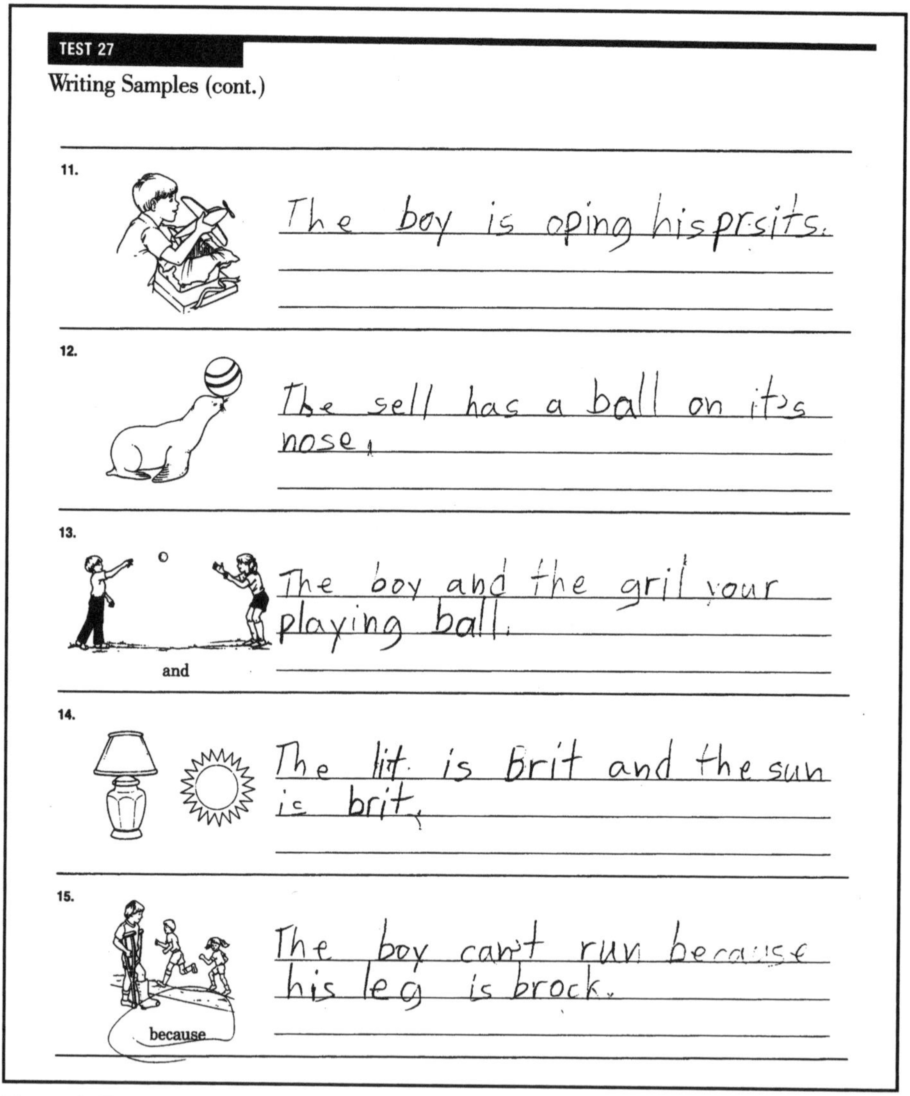

TEST 27

Writing Samples (cont.)

11.

The boy is oping hisprsits.

12.

The sell has a ball on it's nose.

13.

and

The boy and the gril your playing ball.

14.

The lit is brit and the sun is brit.

15.

because

The boy can't run because his leg is brock.

Figure 1.5. Continued.

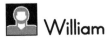 # William

William was referred for evaluation during first grade due to persistent difficulty with reading and spelling skills, as well as a short attention span, hyperactivity, and low frustration tolerance. His early development was described as normal. He had had frequent ear infections as a young child and also had ongoing allergies and mild asthma. Vision and hearing were within normal limits. He received speech therapy at his school to address a mild articulation problem. He also was receiving extra reading assistance at his school, which included some phonics-based instruction. His parents indicated that this was of some benefit. His math skills were described as satisfactory.

Some of William's test scores are shown in Table 1.7. His global intelligence, vocabulary, and visual–motor integration skills were average. Variability in his short-term listening memory skills was evident, with scores ranging from below average to average. He scored average on math tests. His reading scores ranged from low average to average, with mild difficulty being seen in reading fluency and word attack skills for phonetically regular, nonsense words (e.g., *nep, moop*). He scored average on the *Woodcock–Johnson– Revised Tests of Achievement* Dictation and Writing Samples subtests, but below average on the TWS–3. Behavior rating scales completed by his parents and teacher indicated significant symptoms of attention-deficit/hyperactivity disorder (ADHD), combined type.

William's responses on the TWS–3 are shown in Table 1.8, and a page of his responses from the *Woodcock–Johnson–Revised Tests of Achievement* Writing Samples subtest is shown in Figure 1.6. Most of his errors reflect the phonetic stage in spelling development, for example the substitution of *a* for *e* in the words *bed, let,* and *next,* which he wrote as *bad, lat,* and *nat.* Consonant blends usually were represented by a single consonant (e.g., *pat* for *plant, sin* for *spend*). A few transitional misspellings occurred, such as *tow* for *two,* and he was able to use *–ing* correctly at the end of two words (*sining* for *singing, hacing* for *hatching*). My impression was that William displayed mild delays in spelling skills for his age and was at risk for persistent problems, particularly in light of his very low score on the TOPA and history of difficulty with reading in the classroom. The other significant factor was the presence of ADHD symptoms, which also can adversely affect a child's academic performance. On the other hand, there was evidence of recent progress in reading, spelling, and written expression skills.

Additional individualized work was recommended using a phonics-based reading and spelling program, along with explicit training in phonological awareness. His parents had a computer that William enjoyed, and several software programs were suggested. They also planned to obtain a tutor for William during the summer. Behavioral strategies to improve attentional skills in the classroom were discussed. His parents were encouraged to

Table 1.7

Selected Psychoeducational Test Standard Scores for William

	Standard Score
Chronological Age: 7.1	
School Grade: First	
Test Name	
Wechsler Intelligence Scale for Children–3	
Verbal IQ	99
Performance IQ	103
Peabody Picture Vocabulary Test–3	109
Woodcock–Johnson–Revised Tests of Cognitive Ability	
Short-Term Memory	87
Test of Phonological Awareness	73
Bender Visual Motor Gestalt Test	113
Woodcock–Johnson–Revised Tests of Achievement	
Letter–Word Identification	103
Passage Comprehension	104
Word Attack	87
Calculation	98
Applied Problems	108
Dictation	97
Writing Samples	101
Gray Oral Reading Tests–3	88
Test of Written Spelling–3	70

return for a brief reassessment during the first quarter of second grade to update his progress and make further recommendations. My preference would be for William to remain in a regular classroom setting with some instructional modifications and continued assistance through the school supplementary reading program. If this level of support failed to result in satisfactory gains, a special education program might then need to be considered.

Table 1.8

William's Spelling Responses on the *Test of Written Spelling–Third Edition*

Dictated Word	Written Response
stop	stop
bed	bad
let	lat
plant	pat
him	him
went	wit
next	nat
spring	sin
storm	sum
spend	sin
yes	yes
she	seh
us	us
name	nam
two	tow
much	suh
myself	nsaf
people	pelll

36 ✏ Bailet

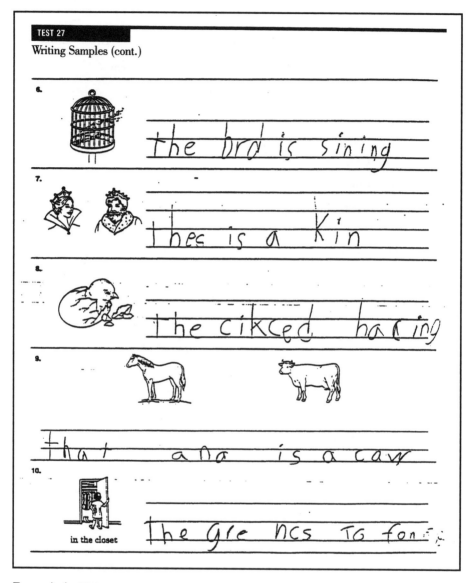

Figure 1.6. Written sentence responses for William near the end of first grade.

References

Adams, M. J., & Henry, M. K. (1997). Myths and realities about words and literacy. *School Psychology Review, 26*(3), 425–436.

Alegria, J., Pignot, E., & Morais, J., Jr. (1982). Phonetic analysis of speech and memory codes in beginning readers. *Memory & Cognition, 10,* 451–456.

Bailet, L. L. (1990). Spelling rule usage among students with learning disabilities and normally achieving students. *Journal of Learning Disabilities, 23*(2), 121–128.

Ball, E. W., & Blachman, B. A. (1991). Does phoneme awareness training in kindergarten make a difference in early word recognition and spelling development? *Reading Research Quarterly, 26,* 46–66.

Beers, J. W. (1980). Developmental strategies of spelling competence in primary school children. In E. H. Henderson & J. W. Beers (Eds.), *Developmental and cognitive aspects of learning to spell: A reflection of word knowledge* (pp. 35–45). Newark, DE: International Reading Association.

Beers, J. W., & Henderson, E. (1977). A study of developing orthographic concepts among first graders. *Research in the Teaching of English, 11*(2), 133–148.

Berko, J. (1958). The child's learning of English morphology. *Word, 14,* 150–177.

Bissex, G. (1980). *Gnys at Wrk: A child learns to write and read.* Cambridge, MA: Harvard University Press.

Blachman, B.A. (1984). Relationship of rapid naming ability and language analysis skills to kindergarten and first-grade reading achievement. *Journal of Educational Psychology, 76,* 610–622.

Boder, E. (1971). Developmental dyslexia: Prevailing diagnostic concepts and a new diagnostic approach. In H. R. Myklebust (Ed.), *Progress in learning disabilities* (Vol. 2, pp. 293–321). New York: Grune & Stratton.

Bradley, L., & Bryant, P. E. (1983). Categorizing sounds and learning to read—A causal connection. *Nature, 301,* 419–421.

Bradley, L., & Bryant, P. E. (1985). *Rhyme and reason in reading and spelling.* (IARLD Monographs No. 1). Ann Arbor: University of Michigan Press.

Bryant, P. E., & Bradley, L. (1980). Why children sometimes write words which they do not read. In U. Frith (Ed.), *Cognitive processes in spelling* (pp. 355–370). London: Academic Press.

Catts, H. W. (1986). Speech production/phonological deficits in reading-disordered children. *Journal of Learning Disabilities, 19*(8), 504–508.

Chomsky, C. (1979). Approaching reading through invented spelling. In L.B. Resnick & P. A. Weaver (Eds.), *Theory and practice of early reading* (Vol. 2, pp. 43–66). Hillsdale, NJ: Erlbaum.

Chomsky, N. (1970). Phonology and reading. In H. Levin & J. Williams (Eds.), *Basic studies in reading* (pp. 3–18). New York: Harper and Row.

Cook, L. (1981). Misspelling analysis in dyslexia: Observation of developmental strategy shifts. *Bulletin of the Orton Society, 31,* 123–134.

Denckla, M. B., & Rudel, R. G. (1976). Rapid "automatized" naming (R.A.N.): Dyslexia differentiated from other learning disabilities. *Neuropsychologia, 14,* 471–479.

Derwing, B. L., & Baker, W. J. (1979). Recent research on the acquisition of English morphology. In R. Fletcher & M. Garman (Eds.), *Language acquisition* (pp. 209–223). Cambridge, England: Cambridge University Press.

Dunn, L. M., & Dunn, L. M. (1997). *Peabody Picture Vocabulary Test–Third Edition.* Circle Pines, MN: American Guidance Service.

Ehri, L. C. (1980). The development of orthographic images. In U. Frith (Ed.), *Cognitive processes in spelling* (pp. 311–338). London: Academic Press.

Ehri, L. C. (1987). Learning to read and spell words. *Journal of Reading Behavior, 19,* 5–31.

Ehri, L. C. (1989). The development of spelling knowledge and its role in reading acquisition and reading disability. *Journal of Learning Disabilities, 22*(6), 356–365.

Ehri, L. C. (1994). Development of the ability to read words: Update. In R. Ruddell, M. Ruddell, & H. Singer (Eds.), *Theoretical models and processes of reading.* Newark, DE: International Reading Association.

Elkonin, D. B. (1973). U.S.S.R. In J. Downing (Ed.), *Comparative reading.* New York: Macmillan.

Felton, R. H., & Wood, F. B. (1989). Cognitive deficits in reading disability and attention deficit disorder. *Journal of Learning Disabilities, 22*(1), 3–13.

Foorman, B. R. (1995). Research on "the great debate": Code-oriented versus whole language approaches to reading instruction. *School Psychology Review, 24*(3), 376–392.

Foorman, B. R., & Francis, D. J. (1994). Exploring the connections among reading, spelling, and phonemic segmentation during first grade. *Reading and Writing: An Interdisciplinary Journal, 6,* 65–91.

Fox, B., & Routh, D. K. (1976). Phonemic analysis and synthesis as word attack skills. *Journal of Educational Psychology, 68,* 70-74.

Fox, B., & Routh, D. K. (1984). Phonemic analysis and synthesis as word attack skills: Revisited. *Journal of Educational Psychology, 76*(6), 1059–1067.

Frith, U. (1979). Reading by eye and writing by ear. In P. A. Kolers, M. Wrolstad, & H. Bouma (Eds.), *Processing of visible language* (pp. 379–390). New York: Plenum Press.

Gerber, M. M. (1984). Investigations of orthographic problem-solving ability in learning disabled and normally achieving students. *Learning Disability Quarterly, 1,* 157–164.

Gerber, M. M., & Hall, R. J. (1987). Information processing approaches to studying spelling deficiencies. *Journal of Learning Disabilities, 20*(1), 34–42.

Gillingham, A., & Stillman, B. (1960). *Remedial training for children with specific disability in reading, spelling and penmanship.* Cambridge, MA: Educators Publishing Service.

Gough, P. B., & Tunmer, W. E. (1986). Decoding, reading, and reading disability. *Remedial and Special Education, 7*(1), 6–10.

Hanna, P. R., Hodges, R. E., & Hanna, J. S. (1971). *Spelling structure and strategies.* Boston: Houghton Mifflin.

Henderson, E. (1990). *Teaching spelling.* Boston: Houghton Mifflin.

Henderson, L., & Chard, J. (1980). The reader's implicit knowledge of orthographic structure. In U. Frith (Ed.), *Cognitive processes in spelling* (pp. 85–116). London: Academic Press.

Hodges, R. E. (1977). *Learning to spell: Theory and research into practice.* Urbana, IL: National Council of Teachers of English.

Invernizzi, M., Abouzeid, M., & Gill, J. T. (1994). Using students' invented spellings as a guide for spelling instruction that emphasizes word study. *Elementary School Journal, 95,* 155–167.

Johnson, D. J., & Myklebust, H.R. (1967). *Learning disabilities: Educational principles and practices.* New York: Grune & Stratton.

Juel, C., & Leavell, J. A. (1988). Retention and nonretention of at-risk readers in first grade and their subsequent reading achievement. *Journal of Learning Disabilities, 21*(9), 571–580.

Katz, R., Shankweiler, D., & Liberman, I. (1982). Memory for item order and phonetic recoding in the beginning reader. *Journal of Experimental Child Psychology, 32,* 474–484.

Klima, E. S. (1972). How alphabets might reflect language. In J. F. Kavanagh & I. G. Mattingly (Eds.), *Language by ear and by eye* (pp. 57–80). Cambridge, MA: MIT Press.

Koppitz, E. M. (1963). *Bender Visual Motor Gestalt Test for Young Children.* Orlando, FL: Grune & Stratton.

Larsen, S. C., & Hammill, D. D. (1994). *Test of Written Spelling–Third Edition.* Austin, TX: PRO-ED.

Liberman, I. Y., Rubin, H., Duques, S. L., & Carlisle, J. (1985). Linguistic abilities and spelling proficiency in kindergartners and adult poor spellers. In D. B. Gray & J. F. Kavanagh (Eds.), *Biobehavorial measures of dyslexia* (pp. 163–176). Parkton, MD: York Press.

Liberman, I. Y., & Shankweiler, D. (1985). Phonology and the problems of learning to read and write. *Remedial and Special Education, 6*(6), 8–17.

Liberman, I. Y., Shankweiler, D., Fischer, F. W., & Carter, B. (1974). Explicit syllable and phoneme segmentation in the young child. *Journal of Experimental Child Psychology, 18,* 201–212.

Lindamood, P., & Lindamood, P. (1998). *The Lindamood phoneme sequencing program for reading, spelling, and speech.* Austin, TX: PRO-ED.

Lundberg, I., Olofsson, A., & Wall, S. (1980). Reading and spelling skills in the first school years, predicted from phonemic awareness skills in kindergarten. *Scandinavian Journal of Psychology, 21,* 159–173.

Luria, A. R. (1973). *The working brain: An introduction to neuropsychology.* New York: Basic Books.

Maclean, M., Bryant, P., & Bradley, L. (1987). Rhymes, nursery rhymes, and reading in early childhood. *Merrill-Palmer Quarterly, 33*(3), 255–281.

Mann, V. A., & Liberman, I. Y. (1984). Phonological awareness and verbal short-term memory. *Journal of Learning Disabilities, 17,* 592–598.

Mann, V. A., Liberman, I. Y., & Shankweiler, D. (1980). Children's memory for sentences and word strings in relation to reading ability. *Memory & Cognition, 8,* 329–335.

Mann, V. A., Tobin, P., & Wilson, R. (1987). Measuring phonological awareness through the invented spellings of kindergarten children. *Merrill-Palmer Quarterly, 33*(3), 365–389.

Marcel, T. (1980). Phonological awareness and phonological representation: Investigation of a specific spelling problem. In U. Frith (Ed.), *Cognitive processes in spelling* (pp. 373–403). London: Academic Press.

Marsh, G., Friedman, M., Welch, V., & Desberg, P. (1980). The development of strategies in spelling. In U. Frith (Ed.), *Cognitive processes in spelling* (pp. 339–353). London: Academic Press.

Moats, L. C. (1983). A comparison of the spelling errors of older dyslexic and second grade normal children. *Annals of Dyslexia, 33,* 121-139.

Moats, L. C. (1995). *Spelling development, disability, and instruction.* Baltimore: York Press.

O'Connor, R. E., Notari-Syverson, A., & Vadasy, P. F. (1996). Ladders to literacy: The effects of teacher-led phonological activities for kindergarten children with and without disabilities. *Exceptional Children, 63*(1), 117–130.

Perfetti, C. A., Beck, I., Bell, L. C., & Hughes, C. (1987). Phonemic knowledge and learning to read are reciprocal: A longitudinal study of first grade children. *Merrill-Palmer Quarterly, 33*(3), 283–319.

Read, C. (1971). Pre-school children's knowledge of English phonology. *Harvard Educational Review, 41*(1), 1–34.

Read, C. (1975). Lessons to be learned from the preschool orthographer. In E. Lenneberg & E. Lenneberg (Eds.), *Foundations of language development* (Vol. 2, pp. 329–346). New York: Academic Press.

Read, C. (1986). *Children's creative spelling.* London: Routledge and Kegan Paul.

Schlagal, R. C. (1989). Constancy and change in spelling development. *Reading Psychology, 10,* 207–232.

Schlagal, R. C. (1992). Patterns of orthographic development in the middle grades. In S. Templeton & D. Bear (Eds.) *Development of orthographic knowledge and the foundations of literacy.* Hillsdale, NJ: Erlbaum.

Schlagal, R. C., & Schlagal, J. (1992). The integrated character of spelling: Teaching strategies for multiple purposes. *Language Arts, 69,* 418–424.

Schwartz, S., & Doehring, D. G. (1977). A developmental study of children's ability to acquire knowledge of spelling patterns. *Developmental Psychology, 13,* 419–420.

Smith, P. T. (1980). Linguistic information in spelling. In U. Frith (Ed.), *Cognitive processes in spelling* (pp. 33–49). London: Academic Press.

Snider, V. E. (1995). A primer on phonemic awareness: What it is, why it's important, and how to teach it. *School Psychology Review, 24*(3), 443–455.

Stanovich, K. (1986). Explaining the variance in reading ability in terms of psychological processes: What have we learned? *Annals of Dyslexia, 35,* 67–96.

Stanovich, K. (1988). Explaining the differences between the dyslexic and the garden-variety poor reader: The phonological-core variable-difference model. *Journal of Learning Disabilities, 21*(10), 590–604.

Stanovich, K. E., Cunningham, A. E., & Cramer, B. B. (1984). Assessing phonological awareness in kindergarten children: Issues of task comparability. *Journal of Experimental Child Psychology, 38,* 175–190.

Stubbs, M. (1980). *Language and literacy: The sociology of reading and writing.* London: Routledge and Kegan Paul.

Tangel, D. M., & Blachman, B. A. (1992). Effect of phoneme awareness instruction on kindergarten children's invented spelling. *Journal of Reading Behavior, 24,* 223–261.

Tangel, D. M., & Blachman, B. A. (1995). Effect of phoneme awareness instruction on the invented spelling of first grade children: A one year follow-up. *Journal of Reading Behavior, 27,* 153–185.

Templeton, S., & Bear, D. R. (Eds.). (1992). *Development of orthographic knowledge and the foundations of literacy: A memorial festschrift for Edmund H. Henderson.* Hillsdale, NJ: Erlbaum.

Torgesen, J. K., & Bryant, B. R. (1994). *Test of Phonological Awareness.* Austin, TX: PRO-ED.

Treiman, R. (1993). *Beginning to spell: A study of first grade children.* New York: Oxford.

Uhry, J. K., & Shepherd, M. J. (1993). Segmentation/spelling instruction as part of a first-grade reading program: Effects on several measures of reading. *Reading Research Quarterly, 28,* 219–233.

Vellutino, F. R., & Scanlon, D. M. (1987). Phonological coding, phonological awareness and reading ability: Evidence from a longitudinal and experimental study. *Merrill-Palmer Quarterly, 33*(3), 321–363.

Venezky, R. L. (1967). English orthography: Its graphical structure and its relation to sound. *Reading Research Quarterly, 2,* 75–105.

Wagner, R. K., & Torgesen, J. K. (1987). The nature of phonological processing and its causal role in the acquisition of reading skills. *Psychological Bulletin, 101*(2), 192–212.

Waters, G. S., Bruck, M., & Seidenberg, M. (1985). Do children use similar processes to read and spell words? *Journal of Experimental Child Psychology, 39,* 511–530.

Wechsler, D. (1991). *Wechsler Intelligence Scale for Children–Third Edition.* San Antonio, TX: Psychological Corporation.

Wiederholt, J. L., & Bryant, B. R. (1992). *Gray Oral Reading Tests–Third Edition.* Austin, TX: PRO-ED.

Woodcock, R. W., & Johnson, M. B. (1989a). *Woodcock–Johnson–Revised Tests of Achievement.* Itasca, IL: Riverside.

Woodcock, R. W., & Johnson, M. B. (1989b). *Woodcock–Johnson–Revised Tests of Cognitive Ability.* Itasca, IL: Riverside.

Spelling Disability in Adolescents and Adults

2

Louisa Cook Moats

Mild to moderate spelling difficulty affects many students in the middle grades and beyond. Like other learning disabilities, spelling disability exists on a continuum of severity. Virtually all people with dyslexia[1] experience significant problems learning to spell (Bruck & Waters, 1988, 1990; Fink, 1998; Fischer, Shankweiler, & Liberman, 1985; Lombardino, Riccio, Hynd, & Pinheiro, 1997; Lyon, 1995; Moats, 1996). The degree of spelling difficulty varies from moderate to severe in individuals who exhibit significant, unexpected problems with word decoding, rapid and accurate word recognition, and fluent reading of connected text. Even if students with reading or language disabilities receive excellent instruction, they often make relatively less progress in spelling than they do in word recognition, word attack, or reading comprehension. Students with the advantages of expert teaching, high IQ, and a good social support system may continue to find spelling a daunting challenge.

Although mild to moderate spelling problems are quite common, teachers often assume that spelling problems cannot be addressed successfully once children are beyond the early grades. Some teachers believe that spelling cannot be taught to older, poor spellers; others assume that children will learn to spell just by reading and writing; and others treat spelling as an unimportant skill that should not take time away from integrated, holistic instruction in writing. Many others would like to teach spelling but are unsure of how to proceed. Too little time seems to be available in the schedules of older students to focus on words. Nevertheless, the worlds of education and employment are much less forgiving of spelling errors than busy teachers may be. Individuals often lose jobs, earn lower grades, or suffer

Note. Louisa C. Moats's work is supported in part by grant number HD 30995.

[1]The term *dyslexia* is used to denote poor decontextualized word reading skills caused by deficiencies in phonological processing; the term has been formally described by the International Dyslexia Association's research committee and explicated in the article by Lyon (1995).

embarrassment if their spelling is poor. Therefore, it behooves us not to ignore this aspect of teaching writing, even if it requires more "technical" knowledge to teach well.

Spelling Is a Linguistic Skill

A research consensus has emerged over the past decade to explain how children learn to read, what differentiates good readers from poor readers, and what can be done to ensure that most children learn to read. The research consensus rests on more than 30 years of programmatic study of reading and related language learning problems (Adams, Treiman, & Pressley, 1998; Fletcher & Lyon, 1998; Snow, Burns, & Griffin, 1998). There has been less focus on spelling, but in the context of reading research, much more is known about the nature and causes of spelling disability than was known 3 decades ago.

Most reading scientists agree that spelling competence is a central linguistic function, not a function dependent on diffuse auditory– or visual– perceptual or memory abilities (Lombardino et al., 1997). Competence in spelling is subsumed by neural networks in the language centers of the brain, and its attainment depends on many of the same linguistic abilities that support reading acquisition (Bruck & Waters, 1990; Ehri, 1989; Lennox & Siegel, 1993). Spelling is an aspect of word knowledge. Word knowledge depends, in turn, on awareness of several layers of language organization, including phonology, sound–symbol correspondences, morphology or word structure, an understanding of word meaning, and sensitivity to the grammatical role of words in sentences (Shankweiler et al., 1995; Templeton & Morris, 1999; Treiman, 1997). Like good readers, good spellers are sensitive to language structure. Poor spellers, on the other hand, are less aware of both oral language structure and the patterns of orthography. This is true no matter what the age of the individual (Lennox & Siegel, 1993; Shankweiler, Lundquist, Dreyer, & Dickinson, 1996). Good spellers are able to use concepts of language to categorize words and organize their mental dictionaries. Poor spellers, on the other hand, do not organize their lexicons with such linguistic logic. The more severe the spelling disorder, the more likely that it can be attributed to faulty phonological, morphological, and orthographic processing (Bruck & Waters, 1990; Moats, 1996; Sawyer, Wade, & Kim, 1999), rather than nonspecific problems of attention, memory, or perception. Before this chapter discusses the characteristics of spelling disabilities, however, it will review the nature of the spelling system and the manner in which most children learn that system, expanding on the information of the previous chapter. The spelling problems of older students are interpretable only within the context of language structure itself, what is known about stages of spelling development, and the psycholinguistic characteristics of individuals with a spelling disability.

Principles of English Spelling: What Must Be Learned

Orthography Is Not a Phonetic Transcription of Speech

As discussed in the previous chapter, English orthography is neither a literal transcription of individual speech sounds nor a phonetic representation of spoken phrases (Chomsky, 1970; Liberman, Shankweiler, & Liberman, 1989). English orthography is morphophonemic; it represents several kinds of information simultaneously, including phonemes (abstract speech sounds), morphemes (the smallest meaningful parts), and the language from which the word came (etymology). To spell the word *opposition* one must know more than its sounds; its structure includes a Latin prefix (op–/ob–), root (*pose*), and a noun suffix (*–ition*), which preempts the silent *e* on the end of *pose*. Meaning, orthographic patterns, and sounds must all be appreciated to spell most words in our language.

At very beginning levels, children learn to spell by sound, generating a symbol for each phoneme. The spelling of this stage is often referred to as "inventive spelling" because the child who is spelling by sound is not aware of the orthographic system. Beyond one-syllable words and regular multisyllabic words, however, sound-symbol correspondence at a surface level is insufficient for spelling English. The reasons are several.

First, real speech is not simply a transparent sequence of separate phonemes. We do not say a sequence of six distinct speech sounds in the word *sprint*, even though the word is, in the abstract, composed of /s/, /p/, /r/, /i/, /n/, and /t/. Words and syllables are undivided segments of speech in which the phonemes are coarticulated—overlapping and welded together. Speech sounds, in reality, blend seamlessly with one another in the spoken word. For example, the consonant blend *nt* in *sprint* is one speech gesture, not two, even though the blend is, in the abstract, two separate phonemes. In addition, the features of each phoneme spread to neighboring phonemes and change them. When we say "educate," the /d/ is pronounced like a /j/, because it is affected by the /yu/ sound that follows it. When we say "congratulate," we pronounce the /t/ like a /ch/, again because it is followed by a /yu/. When we say "seventy," the /t/ is pronounced more like a /d/ than a /t/ by most Americans.

Second, the spelling of English does not represent many of the subtle phonetic changes that occur in naturally spoken words. A readable, learnable orthography must be stable and must represent words more abstractly as meaningful entities. The individual letters in the written word do not, and should not, represent literal phonetic detail. It would not be advantageous to spell *anxious* and *anxiety* differently (Chomsky, 1970), or to spell *differently* without the *e* in *fer,* even though we drop the second vowel in pronunciation.

Letters, letter combinations, and letter sequences represent abstract phonemic segments, syllables, and morphological segments. Therefore, a learner must know the spelling units (letters and letter combinations) used to spell each phoneme and the patterns of letters used to spell speech sound sequences. A good speller will know much more than a literal phonetic transcription of a word. A mature speller will develop awareness of patterns, rules, and meaningful units adopted from Latin and other languages and will know that literal phonetic transcriptions of words in English are often inaccurate. Likewise, an informed teacher will direct students toward the relevant structural features of words during instruction, limiting the directive "sound it out" to those words for which the strategy is truly appropriate.

The Morphological Layer of Written Language

A morpheme is the smallest meaningful unit in the language. It may be a whole word (*condiment*) or a part of a word (*con*scription). Morphemes can be free or stand by themselves without attachment to others (*finger, knead*), or they can be bound to other morphemes and be unable to stand alone as words (*sub-, -ject-, -tion*). Base words may have suffix morphemes classified as inflections (*-ed, -s/es, -ing, -er, -est*), or words may be built through processes of derivation (*con + scrip + tion; pro + scribe; scrip + ture; in + de + scrib + able*). Derivational word building processes involve the addition of prefixes and suffixes to roots that not only alter meaning but that also can change the part of speech: *describe* (v.), *description* (n.), *indescribable* (adj.), *indescribably* (adv.). Spelling of both inflections and derivational morphemes tends to be stable and consistent in English orthography. The plural spelling *-s* can be pronounced as /z/ or /s/, but the spelling of *dogs,* in which the plural is pronounced /z/, uses the letter *s* to signify plurality in spite of the variation of pronunciation.

Abstract similarities between lexical items (words) are often preserved in our orthography, even though derivations of the same word may be pronounced differently. *Social* and *society* are pronounced differently but the consistent spelling of the root *soci* signifies the meaningful relationships among those words. Derivational rules in English often require shifts in either consonant or vowel pronunciations in related words (*electric, electricity, electrical, electrician*). The changes of pronunciation are generated through unconscious, speech production mechanisms of which we may be unaware. Orthography also does not represent the changes of consonant or vowel quality that occur, often by phonological production rule, in spoken words.

To illustrate, the following word pairs all involve consonant shifts: *medical, medicine; precocious, precocity; syntax, syntactic.* Other word pairs involve a change in vowel pronunciation from one form of a word to another, although these follow several different patterns. One pattern involves a change of long vowel to a schwa (/ə/, the unaccented form of many vowels): *incline, inclination; compete, competition; compose, composition.* Another pattern changes a tense (long) vowel to a lax (short) vowel: *profane, profanity; serene, serenity; divine, divinity; cone, conifer.* A third involves alternation of an unstressed vowel (schwa) to a stressed vowel that recovers its identity: *system, systemic; theater, theatrical; image, imagine; mobile, mobility.*

Other complex orthographic patterns preserve meaningful relationships between spoken and written English. These include the preservation of silent letters in the spelling of related lexical items (*oft, often; sign, signal; autumn, autumnal; hymn, hymnal; muscle, muscular*) and the assimilation of prefixes whose pronunciations and spellings change when they are matched to root or base forms (*ad + tend = attend; ad + similate = assimilate; in + mobile = immobile; ad + gressive = aggressive; in + legal + illegal*).

Thus, the relationship between the pronunciation and the spelling of base and derived word forms in English can be linguistically complex (Carlisle, 1987). While the spelling of some derived forms involves no change of pronunciation or spelling of the base word (*fear, fearful; extreme, extremely*), the spelling of other words undergoes changes of varying degrees. Word pairs like *fun–funny, happy–happiness,* and *accuse–accusation,* undergo orthographic changes even though the pronunciation of the base word is constant. (No vowel or consonant pronunciation changes were made in *fun, happy,* or *accuse* to create the derived forms.) Other word pairs such as *electric–electricity* and *public–publicity* undergo a change of pronunciation (phonology) when an ending is added, even though the base form is spelled the same in both the base and its derivation. Still other derived words are characterized by both phonological and orthographic changes, such as *state–statue, precise–precision, flux–fluctuation, consume–consumption.* Furthermore, rules for morphological derivation do not operate consistently or uniformly as words are created for the lexicon. For example, we can have *enjoy* and *enjoyment,* but not *insult* and *insultment.* Certain noun endings just cannot be added to certain words.

Preservation of meaning in a morphophonological spelling system is advantageous for fluent reading: One can directly access meaning by looking at print without having to recode the words into speech (Chomsky, 1970). However, it is far less advantageous for the productive act of spelling. When we spell, the specific letter sequence for a written word may be retrievable only if information about the word's meaning, derivation, grammatical function, and/or linguistic origin is also known. Moreover, the entire letter sequence must be precisely recalled if the word is to be correct. This fact certainly contributes to the dissociation between reading and spelling abilities, evident in the large number of people who can read fluently but who spell poorly. Spelling is more difficult than word recognition in reading.

Later Stages of Learning To Spell

Spelling proficiency develops in a broadly predictable sequence as outlined in Chapter 1. Children's strategies for generating written words change with their developing word knowledge and linguistic awareness. Even though formal spelling instruction may cease in the middle grades of school, adolescents continue to refine their concepts and strategies for spelling through high school (Bear, Invernizzi, Templeton, & Johnston, 1996; Carlisle, 1987; Shankweiler et al., 1996). Students spontaneously revise their strategies for generating unknown words as they learn more words and as they learn how the spelling system is organized (Ehri, 1989; Read, 1986; Treiman, 1997).

The strategies to spell typically employed by students become more varied and responsive to multiple layers of language organization. Young spellers gradually progress from reliance on surface phonetic representation, to more informed use of patterns of sound–symbol relationships, to the incorporation of morphological spelling principles. Beginning at about third or fourth grade, most writers employ "spelling by analogy" strategies. Their mental dictionaries are large enough to allow cross-referencing of new words with words already learned. For example, if a fourth-grader is asked to spell *legislature,* he or she may draw on knowledge of both *legal* and other *–ture* words to understand the spelling. If a sixth grader is asked to spell *anarchy,* he or she may spontaneously think of other known words of similar construction, such as *monarchy.* Words in our mental dictionaries are indexed according to many linguistic features in addition to meaning, including phonetic, phonemic, phonological, graphemic, and morphological segments. Over the entire course of schooling, our knowledge of words is elaborated and deepened so that cross-referencing strategies are possible. For this reason, exposure to print is necessary, but not sufficient, for spelling proficiency to develop in many students. Many aspects of language facility are associated with greater volume of reading and writing (Cunningham & Stanovich, 1997), but learning to spell for many requires deliberate word analysis.

Phonological knowledge continues to develop at least through 10th grade even for normally progressing students. Between fourth and 10th grades, students improve steadily in their ability to spell regular phonological alternation patterns, such as *permit, permission,* or *exclaim, exclamation* (Carlisle, 1987; Templeton & Bear, 1992). If a student has learned the morphological connection between *compose* and *composition,* he or she will more quickly and accurately produce analogous forms such as *impose, impo-*

sition, or *suppose, supposition.* Again, experience with printed words seems to be the source of this increasing ability to generate phonological alternation patterns, because the meaningful similarities among words are more apparent in print than they are in speech, and the vocabulary knowledge required to process morphological relationships is most likely to be learned through extensive reading.

The ability of some students to construct knowledge of linguistic organization in English spelling through exposure to print leads many teachers to the conclusion that spelling is "caught" rather than "taught." Certainly, many students acquire their knowledge through means other than teacher-directed instruction of each individual word. Competent spellers will spontaneously categorize and compare words and extract the pattern redundancies when they see them. So, for example, a good speller, when asked to spell *saturation* may readily spell it like *maturation* or *natural,* without explicitly thinking about the fact that the /t/ spelling before /u/ is pronounced like /ch/. A good speller would know that the phonological pattern of the second syllable is represented by the letter pattern *–ture* and would not make the mistake of spelling the syllable phonetically (*chur*). This analysis may not even be conscious or deliberate. An intuitive grasp of linguistic patterns and correspondences, however, is just what the poor speller lacks.

Older good spellers are also able to access their lexicons or mental dictionaries through several avenues. With intact linguistic processing, students can retrieve words phonologically or orthographically; they can spell words by sound (phonetically) or they can conjure up a spelling pattern. The degree to which these two access routes are independent of one another, however, has been the topic of considerable theoretical debate, with some scientists arguing for a dual-route process, and others arguing that phonological and orthographic processing are more interdependent than separate (Snowling, Goulandris, & Defty, 1996). This theoretical argument is of more than passing interest, because a dual-route model would support the notion that some people can learn to spell "visually," without necessarily being phonologically aware or competent at spelling by sound. The other viewpoint, that these functions are closely amalgamated and interdependent, would suggest that learning both phonology and orthographic structure are necessary for accurate spelling, and that "by-pass" strategies in instruction are not likely to be very effective.

Intact linguistic processing will enable many children to learn individual words with a moderate amount of writing practice, reading practice, and basic instruction in spelling patterns. Normally progressing children do not have to study and memorize every word they eventually write. Poor spellers, on the other hand, seldom generalize word learning to other similar words or patterns unless they are taught explicitly how the system works and when to generalize a rule. Even then, their memory for letter sequences may be unreliable.

Spelling Errors and the Nature of Spelling Disability

Earlier Research on Valid Spelling Error Analyses

The meaning of spelling errors in the diagnosis and treatment of dyslexia and other learning disabilities has been a recurring question addressed in research. A number of recent studies have compared the spellings of older students with dyslexia with those of normally progressing younger students of similar spelling achievement levels (Bruck & Waters, 1990; Carlisle, 1987; Lennox & Siegel, 1993; Moats, 1983; Nelson, 1980; Pennington et al., 1986; Sawyer et al., 1999; Worthy & Invernizzi, 1990). Many of these studies investigated whether the errors of poor spellers were phonetically less accurate than the spellings of normally progressing younger students, and whether there were recurring error patterns that characterized older students with dyslexia. Using structured spelling dictation tasks, researchers have found rather uniformly that error patterns in upper elementary students with spelling disabilities are typical in some ways of early stages of spelling development, and that older poor spellers are in some ways stuck at early levels of spelling development (Frith & Frith, 1983; Worthy & Invernizzi, 1990). For example, they may use letter names to spell parts of words or rely on a sound-by-sound sequential strategy to spell.

The developmental delay hypothesis is unsatisfactory, however, because it does not explain why students fail to progress or why they become stuck with immature spelling strategies. In addition, it does not explain the qualitative problems so evident to teachers, namely, the fact that poor spellers cannot remember the "simple" or high-frequency words needed for writing, that they are unable to proofread effectively, that they confuse similar words, and that they do not retain or generalize well-taught lessons. It also does not explain why the challenges of advanced spelling are never successfully mastered by poor spellers. Poor spellers are puzzling in a number of ways; even if their reading improves after excellent instruction, and they learn formats for written composition, their spelling remains poor in comparison to other language skills.

Phonological Processing Deficits and Poor Spelling

Evidence is substantial that dyslexia involves a core deficit in phonological processing (Felton & Wood, 1989; Liberman et al., 1989; Rack, Snowling, & Olson, 1992; Stanovich & Siegel, 1994), and that poor spellers of all ages do poorly on tests of phonemic awareness, memory for sound sequences, novel word repetition, and other phonological tasks (McDonald & Cornwall, 1995; Rohl & Tunmer, 1988; Stuart & Masterson, 1992). Nevertheless, the presence of phonologically based errors in the writing of students with dyslexia has not been consistently reported by those who have studied error patterns. A common finding in earlier studies has been that older students with dyslexia produce words that are 70% to 80% phonetically accurate, whether whole words or individual sound–spelling units are scored (Moats, 1983; Nelson, 1980; Pennington et al., 1986; Worthy & Invernizzi, 1990). Yet this finding contradicts the general consensus that on tests of phonological processing, individuals with dyslexia do more poorly than normally achieving students at the same level of spelling development.

The contradictory findings regarding the meaning of dyslexic spelling errors and the extent to which they reveal the phonological deficits known to be present in most students with dyslexia suggest that previous or traditional error analysis studies may have missed some of the most important features of older students' difficulties. Several recent studies have approached the analysis of errors differently, and in so doing have begun to expose the fundamental language processing difficulties that students with dyslexia experience (Clarke-Klein & Hodson, 1995; Kibel & Miles, 1994; Moats, 1996; Sawyer et al., 1999; Stage & Wagner, 1992; Viise, 1992).

Phonetic and Phonological Errors Are Not the Same

To learn to read and spell, students must be able to segment, blend, and manipulate the individual phonemes from which words are composed (Ehri & Robbins, 1992; Treiman, 1993). Yet awareness develops unevenly; whole word forms are not gradually brought into focus like a camera lens focusing on an object. Rather, studies of emergent child phonology (Clarke-Klein & Hodson, 1995; Kent, 1992) indicate that phonemes, phoneme combinations, and phonemic contexts in speech production vary in difficulty. For example, pronunciation of the liquids /r/ and /l/, and inclusion of all the consonants in a spoken consonant cluster are later developing than the production of single front consonants. In spelling development, children's attempts at writing reveal their phonological judgments as well as the phonological characteristics of words that are difficult to map to standard orthography (Read, 1986; Treiman, 1993). For example, children's spellings show the ambiguity of tongue flaps in words such as *lidl* (*little*) and the syllabic nature of the final syllable in words such as *badr* (*better*).

Early spelling attempts appear to recapitulate normal phonological processes first evident in children's developing speech production (Hoffman & Norris, 1989), including the systematic simplification, deletion, and substitution of phonemes and syllables. In early speech, children commonly omit consonants from clusters (*chan/train*), interchange voiced and voiceless consonant pairs (*najr/nature*), or substitute front consonants for back ones (*tihn/kitchen*), for example. First-grade children learning to spell often perceive vowel–consonant sequences as indivisible units, especially the sequence of a vowel plus a nasal (*pot/point*) or a vowel plus a liquid (*od/old*)

(Treiman, 1993). Such judgments sometimes show acute sensitivity to phonological reality; those phonemes are coarticulated and are, indeed, difficult to segment because they are abstract, overlapping, and altered in the phonemic context of the whole word. When children learn gradually to identify and spell all the phonemes in English with standard symbols, they do so through successive approximations and the pattern extraction process discussed previously. For older students with dyslexia who are poor spellers, persistent problems occur with those aspects of words that are linguistically difficult at any age.

If dyslexia is a subtle disorder of phonological processing, then the more elusive aspects of phonology should continue to be problematic for students with dyslexia as they acquire literacy (Treiman, 1997). Later developing, complex, or abstract aspects of word learning that involve phonological awareness should present persistent challenges. The phonological system of students with dyslexia may be quite able to handle phonetic recoding at a surface level, or grossly accurate phonetic spelling, but unable to handle the segmentation of phoneme sequences that are most closely amalgamated in speech, such as consonant blends or vowel–liquid combinations in the rime part of the syllable (as in *bird, mold, heard,* or *color*). The student with dyslexia may roughly approximate the number of speech sounds in a written spelling, but may confuse consonants and/or vowels that have similar features, such as the nasals, the liquids, the fricatives, or the back vowels.

Research Evidence for Phonological and Morphological Errors in the Writing of Poor Spellers

Evidence has begun to accumulate that a more linguistically informed approach to error classification does, in fact, uncover some important characteristics of dyslexic spelling. In case study analyses, Moats (1993) found that 90% of a high school student's spelling errors could be classified as representing very specific phonological difficulties. Interestingly, the student had experienced delayed development of speech and chronic misarticulation of /l/ and /r/, and also made a very high proportion of liquid omission and confusion errors in spelling. Viise (1992) studied the orthographic knowledge of adults with low literacy, comparing them to younger students at the same level of achievement. She found that the adults made comparatively more errors on inflections and deleted more unstressed syllables from multisyllabic words. At the same time, the adults' spelling development followed the stage model outlined by Henderson (1990) and his colleagues (Templeton & Bear, 1992). Sawyer et al. (1999) reported that poor readers and poor spellers between ages 10 and 15 are likely to confuse consonants with similar features, especially voicing, and to have difficulty representing all consonants in clusters. Kibel and Miles (1994) reported that consonant clusters, voiced and unvoiced consonant pairs, and later developing speech sounds accounted for a large proportion of the errors demonstrated by upper elementary students.

Other researchers have found a higher incidence of errors involving inflected morphemes in the spelling of middle grade and older children with reading and spelling difficulties (Bailet, 1990; Invernizzi & Worthy, 1989; Worthy & Invernizzi, 1990). Failure to spell inflections, particularly –ed and –s, implies a failure of morphophonemic awareness. These endings are not always syllabic units, although they are morphological entities that are spelled consistently. The –ed looks as if it should be a syllabic unit pronounced with a vowel in the middle. The pronunciation of –ed and –s varies according to the speech sound at the end of the word to which the ending is attached; the –ed may be a /t/ or /d/, as in mocked or dragged, and the –s may be a /s/ or /z/, as in pats or pads. In addition, these endings occur at the ends of words, where they are the least salient in articulation. These apparently simple features are actually very complex. It is logical, then, that they would be difficult for students whose core problem was insensitivity to the phonological, orthographic, and morphophonological structures in spoken and written language (Shankweiler et al., 1996).

A Study of Errors in Spontaneous Writing

To test the hypothesis that the spelling errors of adolescents would, in fact, reveal linguistic deficits if analyzed within linguistic categories more refined than a phonetic or dysphonetic dichotomy (Moats, 1996), I tallied all the spelling errors from the written compositions produced by a group of 19 adolescents with dyslexia who had received intensive remediation for their learning disabilities. The average age of the group was 16. IQs were in the average to superior range for all subjects. After 2 years of intensive teaching, using Orton–Gillingham (Gillingham & Stillman, 1997) methodology, the average spelling achievement in the group was a 5.7 grade equivalent (range 3.4 to 9.8), although the average attainment in word recognition was a 9.3 grade equivalent.

The error categories were derived from previous case studies, the findings of other investigators, the literature on early spelling development, and the literature on phonological characteristics of developing speech. The categories to which errors were assigned were as follows:

I. Orthographic substitutions, or phonologically accurate errors (speech sounds spelled according to identifiable phonetic strategies)

   A. Homophones: by/buy; to/two; then/than

   B. Letter name spellings: opning/opening; reflxs/reflexes; nams/names

   C. Sound-by-sound phonetic spelling: one/own; tipe/type; voly/volley; cind/kind

    D. Failure to change root when ending was added: *haveing/having; easyer/easier*

    E. Student's pronunciation: *resteront/restaurant; ludgery/luxury*

    F. Letter reversals: *emdarase/embarrass*

    G. Plausible schwa misspellings: *attatude/attitude; parants/parents*

    H. Overgeneralization of silent *e*: *plane/plan; lote / lot; hotele / hotel*

II. Phonologically inaccurate spellings

    A. Errors on nasal phonemes

        1. Omission of nasal after a vowel: *kid/kind*

        2. Omission of nasal after a liquid: *leard/learned*

        3. Omission of vowel and nasal: *cling/climbing*

        4. Substitution of one nasal for another: *manber/member*

        5. Omission of entire *–ing* ending: *come/coming*

        6. Insertion of nasal after a vowel: *kinchen/kitchen*

        7. Other: *know/known*

    B. Nasal–liquid substitution: *arould/around*

    C. Errors on liquids /l/ and /r/

        1. Omissions of /l/ before consonants, after vowels: *sefe/self*

        2. Insertion of /l/ or /r/ before a vowel: *wrok/work*

        3. Omission of /r/ after a vowel: *defendo/defenders*

        4. Omission of /l/ or /r/ in a blend: *fends/friends*

        5. Insertion of /r/ or /l/ after a vowel: *cerper/cheaper*

        6. Omission of vowel plus liquid: *evy/every*

        7. Other: *ongus/orange juice*

    D. Omission of nonsonorant consonants

        1. Adjacent consonants across syllable boundaries: *afer/after*

        2. Consonants within clusters: *coot/cost*

        3. Medial syllable-initial: *veio/video*

        4. Word-final: *posity/positive*

    E. Consonant substitutions: *me/be*

F. Consonant additions: *belieft/belief*

G. Vowel substitutions

   1. Stressed vowels: *joib/job*

   2. Unstressed vowels: *resions/reasons*

   3. *R*-controlled vowels: *werey/worry*

H. Deletion of schwa: *manged/managed*

I. Whole syllable or stressed syllable deletion: *Colordo/Colorado*

J. Sequence is confused: *lost/lots*

K. Word substitutions: *close/cost*

L. Multiple errors, undecipherable: *protilly/prosperity*(?)

III. Morphophonological misspellings

  A. Morphophonological errors on *–ed*

    1. Omit *–ed*: *talk/talked*

    2. Phonetic spelling of *–ed*: *helpet/helped; hapend/happened*

    3. Addition of *–ed*: *affectived/effective*

    4. Other: *spstow/supposed to*

  B. Morphophonological errors on *–s*

    1. Plural /s/ on nouns omitted: *goal/goals*

    2. Verb/adverb markers omitted: *ski/skis*

    3. Contractions with /s/ for *is: that/that's*

    4. Additions of noun/verb inflections: *teachers/teacher; leves/leave*

    5. Other: *reasond / reasons*

The 19 subjects demonstrated widely varying problems with spelling. As would be expected, phonological, morphophonological, and orthographic errors were most frequent in the students with the lowest spelling scores. Phonological spelling accuracy did not vary with IQ in this sample; the brightest subject was also the most impaired in spelling. IQ was not a factor in how fast the students progressed in spelling over a 2-year span.

The students fell roughly into two groups: those with achievement in spelling at or above the sixth-grade level, after intensive remediation, and those who remained below the sixth-grade level. The poorer spellers made more than three times as many errors per 100 words as the better spellers. The spelling errors made by the poorer spellers were almost twice as likely to involve phonological and morphophonological inaccuracies. In the more improved students, only 26% of the errors were phonologically or morphologically inaccurate; in the less improved, lower achieving students, 46% of all the errors they made were attributable to faulty phonological processing. Of those phonologically inaccurate errors in the lower achieving group, 24% were specific to nasal and liquid speech sounds. The largest proportion of the nasal and liquid errors occurred on speech sounds that came after a vowel and before a consonant. The speech sound /n/ was much more commonly misspelled than /m/, however.

Another 23% of the body of errors in the poorest spellers' compositions involved omissions, substitutions, and confusions of inflections –ed and –s. These errors were very uncommon in the compositions of the students who progressed beyond a sixth-grade spelling achievement level.

The lowest achievers made much slower progress in spelling over the 2-year instructional period. Their average rate of gain was 1.4 years in spelling achievement. In the group who achieved at a higher level, who also were more accurate at phonological representations, the average rate of gain was 2.5 years for 2 years of instruction.

The most commonly misspelled words were high-frequency words that often have unusual spellings: *their/there, your/you're, too/to, want, buy, friend, when, where, were, really, know, every,* and *because.* Other commonly misspelled sight words included *something, than/then, would, which, what, until, through, some, other, of, my, from,* and *do.*

The spontaneous misspellings of these adolescents suggested that those with the most intractable spelling problems did indeed make a high number of errors attributable to incomplete or faulty phonological and morphological processing. The poorest achievers differed from those with milder problems in the proportion and nature of phonologically based errors. The poorest spellers often produced grossly accurate phonetic spellings, but they nevertheless had marked and persistent difficulties with specific linguistic constructions. These included segments that were linguistically ambiguous or complex and speech sounds that were hard to detect in the spoken word. Unaccented vowels, consonant blends, liquid and nasal phonemes after vowels, and phonemes that are easily mistaken for others were among the most commonly misspelled elements. Inflections –ed and –s continued to be problematic.

 Case Example 1

The story about cave men in Figure 2.1 was written by a 16-year-old, well-educated girl whose verbal IQ measured in the superior range (120). She had struggled with dyslexia all her life, but with persistence and tutoring help, she had learned to read at grade level when tests were untimed. She was not inhibited about expressing her ideas in writing, although she was continually frustrated by her inability to recall spellings.

This subject is unusual in that she spells almost all of the past tense and plural inflections correctly, except *sink/skinned* and *passd/passed*. However, her problems with phoneme identification, sequencing, and representation are notable. Blends that include an /l/ or /r/ are difficult (*theroing/throwing; thoing/throwing; colthes/clothes*) as are other blends (*sink/skinned*) and r-controlled vowels (*frist/first*). She omits the medial sonorant from *mammoths* (*maothe*). She spells some words with an immature phonetic strategy (*famly/family; hungre/hungry*) and makes two errors on consonant digraph spellings (*togeter/together; flase/flesh*) that would be atypical even for a second- or third-grader.

This student, in spite of her success in reading, would benefit from an intensive approach designed to help her identify, sequence, and spell all the phonemes in one-syllable words, such as *The Lindamood Phoneme Sequencing Program for Reading, Spelling, and Speech* (Lindamood & Lindamood, 1998)

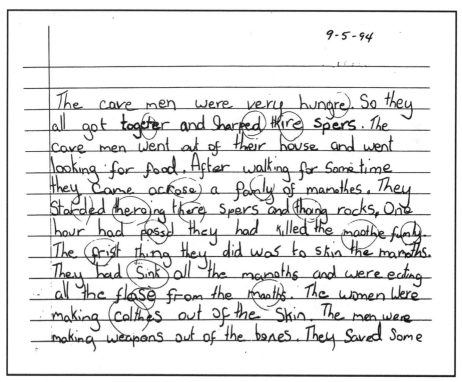

Figure 2.1. Composition of 15-year-old dyslexic girl.

or the *Wilson Language Program* (Wilson, 1996). If she does not learn to identify, separate, sequence, or blend speech sounds, spelling will be very difficult.

Case Example 2

This 12-year-old boy (BH) is extremely bright but struggled with reading as
a first-grader. After appropriate remediation, he learned to read and by second grade was "on track" with reading. His teachers often commended his
imaginative, descriptive writing. His spelling, however, was less responsive
to remediation, and by sixth grade was quite poor in relation to grade-level
expectations. In addition, his expository writing indicated inadequate mastery of syntax, paragraph, and discourse structure. At that point, his family
sought intensive help for his persistent phonological and linguistic processing weaknesses. As an initial screening, a qualitative inventory of spelling
development was administered (see Figures 2.2a, 2.2b, and 2.2c).

BH overrelied on immature sound-by-sound strategies to spell, but had not
internalized the rules, patterns, and morphological structures in orthography
that depend on deeper awareness of language. His errors in written expression,
as well as the spelling inventory errors, included many good phonetic spellings
that showed limited memory for the specific letter sequences in words:

smuge/smudge	abilitys/abilities	riesadent/resident
traped/trapped	feaver/fever	macinery/machinery
wazing/waxing	pennys/pennies	lessen/lesson
cogratilated/ congratulated	distence/distance	discovory/discovery
	anserd/answered	waring/wearing

Although his spelling was quite easy to read because of its surface phonetic
accuracy, BH demonstrated subtle weaknesses on tests of phonological processing that required him to segment, identify, and manipulate four or five
speech sounds within one syllable. Multisyllabic words also were processed
inaccurately. As with many "phonetically accurate" good readers and poor
spellers, the underlying phonological problem was subtle, and the more obvious deficits were with complex letter-pattern awareness (*smuge/smudge*); use
of orthographic ending rules (*traped/trapped; pennys/pennies*); and awareness of morphology (*cogratilated/congratulated*). Remediation with phoneme
tracking activities and multisyllabic word analysis sharpened his perception
of sounds and syllables; subsequently, he was better able to recall orthographic sequences. Intensive study of language structure and writing skills
for several hours per day during a summer session helped BH improve significantly.

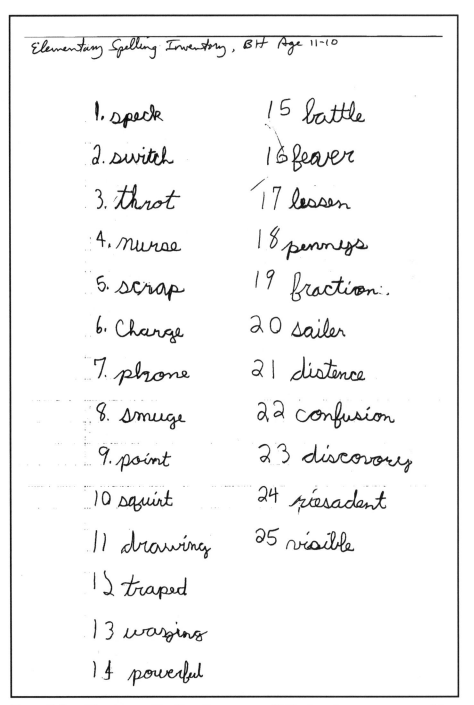

Elementary Spelling Inventory, BH Age 11-10

1. speck
2. switch
3. throt
4. nurse
5. scrap
6. Charge
7. phone
8. smuge
9. point
10 squirt
11 drawing
12 traped
13 wasing
14 powerful

15 battle
16 feaver
17 lessen
18 penneys
19 fraction.
20 sailer
21 distence
22 confusion
23 discovery
24 presadent
25 visible

Figure 2.2a. Elementary Spelling Inventory of BH when he was 11 years old.

(Handwritten notes on sheet: "age 11 yrs. 10 mos.", "Grade 5", "he categorized it")

Elementary Spelling Inventory—Individual Score Sheet

Grade 5 Date _____ Total Pts _____

	Short vowel	Blend/ digraph	Long vowel	Other vowel	Complex consonant	inflection	Syllable juncture	Unaccented syllable	suffix	Correct	Word Totals
1. speck	e ✓	sp ✓			ck ✓					✓✓	4
2. switch	i ✓	sw ✓			tch ✓					✓	4
3. throat			oa		thr ✓					✓	2
4. nurse				ur ✓							1
5. scrape			a-e		scr ✓					✓	4
6. charge		ch ✓		ar ✓	ge ✓					✓	3
7. phone		ph ✓	o-e ✓							✓	2
8. smudge	u ✓	sm ✓			dge						3
9. point		nt ✓		oi ✓							3
10. squirt		squ ✓		ir ✓						✓	3
11. drawing		dr ✓		aw ✓		-ing ✓				✓	4
12. trapped		tr ✓				-pped				✓	2
13. waving						-ving					0
14. powerful				ow ✓				-er ✓	-ful ✓	✓✓	4
15. battle							tt ✓	-tle ✓		✓	3
16. fever							v ✓	-er ✓		✓	3
17. lesson							ss ✓	-on			1
18. pennies						-ies	nn ✓				2
19. fraction									-tion ✓		
20. sailor							l ✓		-or	✓	2
21. distance							st ✓		-ance		
22. confusion									-sion ✓		2
23. discovery								dis-	-ery		
24. resident								si	-dent ✓	✓	
25. visible									-ible ✓		1
Feature Totals	3	9	1	6	5	1	6	4	5	14	Total Pts 54

(Note in inflection column, row 5: "ai ?")

Figure 2.2b. Elementary Spelling Inventory—Individual Score Sheet that shows the scoring of the inventory in Figure 2.2a (F. Johnston, personal communication, 1998).

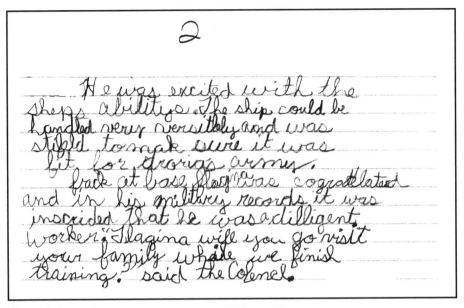

Figure 2.2c. Writing sample to assess BH's spelling.

Guidelines for Assessment of Older Students

Thorough assessment of dyslexia or language-based learning disabilities should include at least a measure of spelling achievement on a dictated word list, a developmental spelling inventory, and an analysis of errors in both dictation and spontaneous writing. Older students' strategies for handling spelling problems during writing should be observed as well. Does the student limit word choices in writing to those he or she can spell? Does the student fail to recognize incorrect spellings? Does the student misspell common, high-frequency words? Does the student fail to apply what he or she has learned under conditions of supervised teaching and practice? All of these characteristics are common with students who have intrinsic difficulties with written language processing (dyslexia and related language learning disorders). Students with other kinds of learning disorders, including those related to attention-deficit disorder, may also be weak in spelling, but they are unlikely to make errors of phonological confusion or to be as poor as students with dyslexia on dictated tests (Lombardino et al., 1997).

Spelling achievement levels should be assessed with a well-normed, representative list of single words that progress in difficulty. The *Kaufman Test of Educational Achievement* (Kaufman & Kaufman, 1985), the *Wide Range Achievement Test* (Jastak & Wilkinson, 1984), and the *Test of Written*

Spelling–Fourth Edition (TWS–4) (Larsen, Hammill, & Moats, 1999) are among the possibilities (see reviews in Chapter 7). The TWS–4 was recently redesigned into a stronger measure than its predecessors. The Predictable and Unpredictable word lists of earlier editions were consolidated into one list, and alternate forms were created to support pretesting and posttesting.

A qualitative inventory of spelling development is a useful tool for measuring acquisition of specific phoneme–grapheme, syllable, and morpheme correspondences as they exist in real words. In use for almost 2 decades at the McGuffey Reading Center at the University of Virginia, developmental spelling inventories were developed by Edmund Henderson (1990) and his graduate students (Bear et al., 1996; Ganske, 2000a, 2000b). A qualitative inventory of spelling development is an efficient and effective way to group children for spelling instruction. An inventory consists of word lists that use progressively more complex and advanced correspondences and that reflect the order in which orthographic knowledge is typically acquired.

Several versions of developmental inventories exist, but each is based on the valid theory that spelling knowledge accumulates in a predictable sequence from simpler linguistic constructions to more complex ones. Lists progress from words with single-syllable, highly predictable spellings, to single-syllable words with more complex (but still predictable) graphemes, to regular syllable patterns and their combinations, to words with Latin and Greek morphological structure.

Of course, spelling ability should be assessed in relation to decoding skills (single-word real and nonword reading), reading fluency, reading comprehension, phonological processing, syntax comprehension, and composition.

Spelling Instruction with Adolescents and Adults

Spelling improvement can occur in older poor spellers if it is carried out systematically over a long period of time. Individuals with significant phonological or language-based disorders seldom progress in spelling as fast as they can improve in reading. Although the ultimate gains may be modest, they may be sufficient for a person who can then use proofreading aides. An effective instructional program for poor spellers will be integrated with other language instruction and will be characterized by:

- direct teaching with frequent teacher–student interaction and a high response rate during instruction
- controlled introduction of new linguistic information
- modeling and immediate feedback during writing

- linking of listening, speaking, reading, and writing
- systematic, sequential, and cumulative teaching of sounds, syllables, and morphemes
- daily, sustained writing practice

Teacher-Directed, Systematic Practice with Controlled Amounts of New Information

The term *systematic* in spelling instruction means that patterns of correspondence in English orthography are emphasized in the lesson design, and they are presented in a logical order. Instruction proceeds step-by-step, providing sufficient practice with concepts and patterns already taught in previous lessons. Thus, systematic teaching is also cumulative and redundant. The teacher assumes that students will forget, even as they study, and that some students need a great deal of practice before associations and concepts are internalized. Instruction is carried out with the aid of careful record keeping to determine when words, patterns, and concepts are learned.

Why is it necessary to be systematic? First, our orthography is a system of correspondences that are predictable by rule and pattern (Henry, 1993, 1999; Moats, 2000); second, students are more likely to learn the system if they receive organized, sequential practice. Many students will not remember the spelling of words simply from reading them or from writing them occasionally, on an "as needed" basis. Spelling requires explicit and precise recall of orthographic sequences and many examples of a pattern should be presented at once. In addition, many of the most commonly used words in English are of Anglo-Saxon origin and have retained low-frequency or odd spellings that also must be memorized through repeated, correct use in writing.

Regardless of the content, people with dyslexia or spelling disabilities generally learn better when the amount to be learned is controlled, the amount of practice is monitored, and reinforcement is liberally given (Lyon & Moats, 1988). To build up word images in memory and to ensure that words are so well learned that they can be recalled without delay or extra attention, a great deal of practice of a few elements at a time is required. A good rule of thumb is 80% old information, 20% new information in a lesson plan designed for a person who spells poorly.

Limit the Number of Words

The number of words presented at one time also needs to be limited for students with spelling disabilities. Reith et al. (1974) found that poor spellers recalled more words by the end of the week if they learned five or six a day and were tested on those daily. Good spellers, however, learned well with all 20 words given on Monday. Bryant, Drabin, and Gettinger (1981) found that students with severe spelling disabilities did best with only three new words a day. These data are most applicable to situations when students are trying to memorize specific words.

When students are being taught a concept, rule, or generalization about sound–symbol correspondence, such as the "*f, l, s* doubling rule," only one concept or pattern should be taught at a time. However, ample practice with 30 or more examples in one lesson is often necessary for the redundant pattern to be internalized. Students learn patterns through repeated attention to the relevant features of many examples. Poor spellers need more experience with print and more focus and repetition than good spellers.

Modeling and Immediate Feedback

With poor spellers, effective teaching also entails direct instruction and much interaction between student and teacher. Activities such as quiet completion of worksheets and looking at words on flash cards until they can be written from memory do not result in useful learning, especially for older students who must "unlearn" some bad habits. Students should be asked to write words and sentences to dictation and then receive immediate corrective feedback from the teacher, who might use an overhead projector to proofread sentences with a group. Error imitation and modeling of word analysis and correction (Nulman & Gerber, 1984) has been validated as a strategy for teaching students with learning disabilities. The teacher reproduces the student's error and then corrects it, explaining the difference between the incorrect and correct words, before asking the student to write the word correctly.

Multisensory Instruction

The term *multisensory* refers to the simultaneous engagement of hearing, seeing, saying, and feeling during spelling practice. The initials VAKT—Visual, Auditory, Kinesthetic, Tactile—refer to multisensory instruction of basic language skills. Students might be asked to say a word while writing it with fingers on a rough surface, or might be asked to say a word slowly, segment its sounds while tapping fingers for each sound, say the letters that correspond to the sounds, and write them. Although it is not entirely clear from research why multisensory techniques are most efficacious with children with dyslexia, experienced remedial teachers have recommended them for decades (e.g., Birsh, 1999; Carreker, 1999; Fernald, 1943; Gillingham & Stillman, 1997).

One likely reason for the efficacy of the multisensory approach is that it encourages the student to externalize and focus upon the phonemic elements of the word by saying it slowly and deliberately, noticing how each phoneme is represented. This activity facilitates the comparator function, the active differentiation of similar word forms and conscious matching of sound to symbol, viewed as central to spelling by Lindamood, Bell, and Lindamood (1992). Moreover, more attention is deployed when several sensory modalities are engaged simultaneously, probably resulting in increased brain activation levels and increased chances for information storage.

Systematic, Sequential, Cumulative Instruction

Individuals who are poor spellers are insensitive to the structure of spoken and written language. They need much more practice than good spellers to remember sound–symbol associations. They do not spontaneously perceive the semantic, phonological, or orthographic relationships among words that are part of a derivational network. When the correspondences, syllable patterns, and other redundancies of the language are presented one at a time in a logical sequence, the elements are differentiated, brought into focus, and related to one another. All the elements are not equally difficult, and repetition of the hardest concepts and associations can be built into lessons as needed. The approximate sequence of spelling instruction is as follows:

Sequence of Spelling Instruction

1. Explicit practice with phoneme identification and segmentation

2. Association of symbols with sounds

3. Identification, segmentation, and combination of phonemes in one-syllable word patterns

4. Identification, analysis, and writing of inflections

5. Conditional within-word patterns

6. Homophones

7. Orthographic change rules when endings are added

8. Syllabication and the juncture of syllables

9. Latin and Greek morphemes and morpheme combination

Early Introduction of Inflections

As soon as students are reading and writing verb forms, they are ready to be introduced to the past tense –ed morpheme. As soon as they are reading and writing noun forms, they are ready to learn the plural –s spelling. Learning that these morphemes are spelled consistently in spite of variations in pronunciation is the first step to realizing that spelling represents meaning, often in preference to sound. Explicit teaching of the past tense necessitates identification of the /d/, /t/, or /ed/ that ends words such as *begged, walked,* and *wanted,* before words are written to dictation. Inflection spellings should be reviewed and practiced often for many years. It is insufficient to present one lesson on each and expect the learning to be internalized.

Conditional Word and Syllable Patterns

Many patterns and generalizations are predictable but conditional. They include the spellings of *tall, annoy, glue, glove,* and *most.* In these cases, the student can be asked either to understand a pattern from examples (inductive learning) or to apply a given rule or principle to examples (deductive learning). The inductive approach is a powerful tool for bright students who enjoy solving puzzles. It is illustrated by the following exercise to teach the *ch, tch* generalization:

Given this list of words,

inch	march	botch
starch	pooch	kitchen
pitch	bunch	butcher
hatchet	fetch	pinch
catch	ranch	stitch
pouch		

discover when *tch* is used to spell /ch/ at the ends of words or syllables.

Students should be told there are a few exceptions, including *rich, much, such, which, attach, sandwich,* and *bachelor.* A word sort activity (Bear et al., 1996) for discovering patterns can be carried out with words on cards.

If the inductive approach is confusing or ineffective with students because they are unable to see the patterns in the examples, then a deductive approach must be taken. A deductive approach calls for the teacher to state the rule and ask the student(s) to apply it to examples. With the word list above, the teacher might state, "A one-syllable word ending in /ch/ spells it *tch* after an accented short vowel. In all other cases, /ch/ is spelled *ch.*" Then words could be grouped, read, and spelled to dictation.

Homophones

Their, there, and *they're; you're* and *your; its* and *it's* are among the most often misspelled words in the language. Other spellings of words that sound the same but differ in meaning and spelling, such as *course* and *coarse, knight* and *night, prophet* and *profit* are commonly confused by students who cannot rely on letter memory. The best one can hope for in cases of very poor spellers is to clarify confusions among words they use most often, because practice in context is what eventually develops the correct word habit.

Teachers often claim it takes an entire year of repeated practice to straighten out *there/their/they're* confusion in older students. Matching games in which spelling and meaning are paired are helpful, at least in sensitizing the writer to what must be looked up, along with dictated phrases given regularly. A comprehensive list of homophones can be found in *The New Reading Teacher's Book of Lists* (Fry, Fountoukidis, & Polk, 1985). Recall is facilitated when the words are used repeatedly in phrases, sentences, cloze exercises, analogies, jokes, cartoons, and puns. Homophones should be taught a few at a time; however, only the most able learners can work with the long lists that often appear in workbooks.

Syllable Patterns and Syllable Juncture

The syllable should be defined as a pronounceable unit that always contains a vowel sound and a vowel letter (exceptions *rhythm; –ism*). Children with spelling difficulties benefit from learning the six syllable types (see Table 2.1).

One reason for teaching syllables is that redundant patterns in longer words can be much more quickly discerned. Another reason is that the rules for adding endings to words and the way in which syllables are combined into longer words depend on the type of syllable(s) in the word. Finally, spellings become more predictable when the type of syllable is taken into account. For example, the most common spelling of long *a* in an open syllable within a multisyllable word (*radio, vacation, stable*) is simply the letter *a*, and not the other seven alternatives.

If one knows about syllable types and syllable division, one can remember more easily that *dinner* has two *n*s and *diner* has one. In *dinner,* the first vowel is short, the first syllable is closed by an *n*, and another *n* separates the first vowel from the second. Most commonly, a short-vowel (closed) syllable is separated from the vowel of a following syllable by two intervening consonants. A double *n* is necessary in words like *beginning* because the second syllable is closed and the double letter protects the short *i* vowel sound when the *–ing* is added. There are many excellent programs for teaching syllable structure to older students including *Scientific Spelling* (Carreker, 1992);

Table 2.1
Six Syllable Types

Syllable Type	Characteristics
Closed *rab bit* *bed bug* *bas ket* *pic nick ing*	These syllables contain a single-letter, short vowel followed by a consonant. In a multisyllable word, a short vowel is usually protected by two consonants. Thus, if a short vowel is heard in the first syllable, there are most likely two consonants between it and the next vowel.
Open *moment* *mutation* *decide*	An open syllable ends with a long vowel spelled with a single vowel letter. The long vowel in an open syllable is usually separated from the next syllable with only one consonant letter or no consonant.
R-controlled *worthy* *server* *nurture* *endorse* *starboard*	When a vowel is followed by /r/, the vowel loses its identity as a long or short vowel. It is coarticulated with the /r/, so much so that, in the case of /er/, there is no separable vowel and consonant. A similar phenomenon occurs when /l/ follows a vowel. There is a set of *r*-controlled vowel spellings children must learn through practice with many examples.
Vowel Team *about* *repeat* *embroil* *apiece*	Many long vowels are spelled with two vowel letters working as a team, such as *ai, ay, ee, ea, ie, oa,* and *ue.* Diphthongs are also spelled with two letters: *oi, oy, ou.* The letter *w* can work as part of a vowel team (*aw, ew, ow*) even though it is never a vowel by itself. These teams, which are difficult for many poor spellers, can appear at the middle or end of words or before certain consonants (e.g., *aw* before /n/ and /l/).
Vowel–Consonant–*e* *compete* *reside* *milkshake*	In the vowel–consonant–silent *e* pattern, the vowel sound is long, there is one intervening consonant, and the *e* is silent. The silent *e* can be removed when a suffix is added that begins with a vowel, as in *competing, refutable, residence.*
Consonant-*le* *bugle* *juggle* *little* *rifle*	When the syllabic /l/ sound occurs at the ends of spoken words, it is often preceded by a consonant that is part of the last syllable. Thus in the word *bugle,* the first syllable is open and the second is a consonant–*le* combination. In the word *little,* the first syllable is closed, and the second is a consonant–*le.*

Language! Level II (Greene, 1995); *Patterns for Reading and Spelling* (Henry & Redding, 1996); *Megawords* (Johnson & Bayrd, 1983); and the *Wilson Language Program* (Wilson, 1996).

Latin and Greek Morpheme Patterns

Latin-based words are usually taught after basic Anglo-Saxon vocabulary has been learned (Henry, 1993). In some ways they are easier to spell than Anglo-Saxon words. They do not use the problematic digraphs so common in Anglo-Saxon spellings, and because many spellings are meaning-based prefixes, roots, and suffixes, they tend to be constant even though many are reduced to schwa when they are unaccented. If students learn to recognize those meaningful units, many spellings will seem more logical. For example, *recommend* does not have two *c*s because the prefix *re–* is added to the root *commend*. The morpheme often maintains its integrity in spelling.

There is ample evidence from cognitive psychology that words sharing derivational relationships should be taught together (Moats & Smith, 1992; Templeton & Morris, 1999). Many roots of Latin origin have consonants whose phonetic form changes in derived words such as the /t/, /c/, and /s/ that appear in *partial, magician,* and *confusion.* In addition, reduced vowels can be ambiguous in various derived forms (*confidence, sedative, competition*). In many words with ambiguous vowels or chameleon consonants, the correct spelling of a base word or derivation can be recovered more easily if it is learned in partnership with a word sharing the same root and more transparent pronunciation.

On any list of hard-to-spell words, there are some that can be taught so that root-derivative relationships are made clear: *differ, different; favor, favorite; child, children; autumn, autumnal; sign, signal; resign, resignation; vacate, vacation; athlete, athletic; theatre, theatrical; magic, magician.*

Many other words that turn up on hard-to-spell lists are rule-based or comprise affix–root constructions that make the spelling make sense. There is no reason why *beneficial, advice, attend,* or *misspell* should be learned in isolation as sight words, when all have prefixes. The method for teaching such words should call attention to the word's structure at the levels of sound, syllable, and meaningful parts.

Greek Patterns

Words of Greek origin comprise a large segment of our scientific vocabulary and are best studied in the context of science and math. The spellings of *y* for /i/ (*gym, sphinx, syllable, krypton*), *ph* for /f/ (*photo, sphere, graph*), and *ch* for /k/ (*chorus, chameleon, ache*) are Greek derivatives. Greek words combine morphemes but assign them equal status, like English compounds (*stratosphere, phonograph, thermometer*). The spellings tend to be very consistent and phonically transparent, and thus easier than words from other languages. Programs that teach Greek roots are the *Language! Roots* supplement to *Language!* (Bebko, Alexander, & Doucet, 1997) and *Patterns for Reading and Spelling* (Henry & Redding, 1996).

About Ending Rules

The three major rules requiring an orthographic change when endings are added to words seem daunting for students to learn and frustrating for teachers to teach (see Table 2.2 for ending rules.)

Ending rules must be presented at intervals over several years, along with repeated reinforcement when corrective feedback about spelling is given. Consistent practice is needed rather than one or two lessons. Furthermore, these rules should be introduced after students have the conceptual underpinnings: a firm grasp of single-syllable spellings; the concepts of consonant, vowel, and syllable; and the ability to read multisyllabic words.

The internalization of orthographic change rules is very difficult for many poor spellers. Students with spelling disabilities will often fail to notice when a rule should be applied, even if they know the rule (Carlisle, 1987; Liberman, Rubin, Duques, & Carlisle, 1985; Shankweiler et al., 1996). Poor spellers will often recall specific word spellings without evidence that they have internalized or automated the rule that governs them. These students often end up relying on a personal list of learned words that constricts their writing considerably.

Additional Strategies To Aid Memorization

Several additional strategies for spelling instruction can be helpful when employed selectively and sensibly.

1. *Invoke a "spelling pronunciation."* This works well for words with silent letters and foreign or irregular spellings that do not match pronunciation, such as *Wednesday, was,* and *antique.*

2. *Group words with like, but unusual, spelling–meaning patterns.*

two	one	there	their
twenty	once	here	heir
twelve	only	where	

3. *Employ mnemonic devices (association links).* He **meant** to be **mean**. There's **a rat** in sep**arat**e. Knights would **die val**iantly in me**dieval** times. **Loose** as a **goose**. It's hard to **lose** your **nose**. **Sally** finally came home.

Table 2.2
Orthographic Rules for Adding Suffixes to Roots or Base Words

1a. The doubling rule: When a one-syllable word with one vowel ends in one consonant, double the final consonant before adding a suffix beginning with a vowel.

Examples: *running, batter, gunned, wettest*

1b. The advanced doubling rule: When a word has more than one syllable, double the final consonant when adding an ending beginning with a vowel, if the
final syllable is accented and has one vowel followed by one consonant.

Examples: *conferring, conference; occurrance, occurred; opening, beginning*

2. The silent *e* rule: When a root word ends in a silent *e*, drop the *e* when adding a
suffix beginning with a vowel. Keep the *e* before a suffix beginning with a consonant.

Examples: *confining, wasteful, extremely, excitement, hoping, spicy*

3. The *y* rule: When a root word ends in a *y* preceded by a consonant, change the *y*
to *i* before a suffix, except *–ing*. If the root word ends in a *y* preceded by a
vowel, just add the suffix.

Examples: *studying, studious, happier, monkeying, jellied, beautiful, crying*

4. *Highlight visual–orthographic features of words.* People with poor orthographic memory may store and retrieve word images more readily if novelty or
contrast is used to highlight letter sequences. Techniques that may be useful
include color coding (to contrast vowels and consonants); underlining; using different fonts on a word processor; writing letters in different sizes; or instructing
the student to create a mental image around the letters of a word. The effectiveness of these manipulations, however, is not well researched at present.

Conclusion

Older students who are poor spellers can be taught, although their progress
may be slow. Learning to spell is one of the most challenging of all linguistic
skills. Methods that work, however, are those that provide insight into the
structure of language through a logical, sequential, linguistically informed
approach. Instructional methods will depend upon the nature of the vocabulary to be learned, the developmental level of the students, and the types of
learning difficulties they may present. The goal of spelling instruction, in
summary, is to enhance the students' understanding of word structure and
their ability to use words fluently and accurately in their writing.

References

Adams, M. J., Treiman, R., & Pressley, M. (1998). Reading, writing, and literacy. In I. E. Sigel & K. A. Renninger (Eds.), *Handbook of child psychology, Fifth Edition: Child psychology in practice* (Vol. 4, pp. 275–355). New York: Wiley.

Bailet, L. L. (1990). Spelling rule usage among students with learning disabilities and normally achieving students. *Journal of Learning Disabilities, 23,* 121–128.

Bear, D. R., Invernizzi, M., Templeton, S., & Johnston, F. (1996). *Words their way: Word study for phonics, vocabulary, and spelling instruction.* Englewood Cliffs, NJ: Merrill.

Bear, D. R., & Templeton (1998). Explorations in developmental spelling: Foundations for learning and teaching phonics, spelling, and vocabulary. *The Reading Teacher, 52,* 222–242.

Bebko, A., Alexander, J., & Doucet, R. (1997). *Language! Roots.* Longmont, CO: Sopris West.

Birsh, J. (Ed.) (1999). *Multisensory teaching of basic language skills.* Baltimore: Brookes.

Bruck, M., & Waters, G. (1988). An analysis of the spelling errors of children who differ in their reading and spelling skills. *Applied Psycholinguistics, 9,* 77–92.

Bruck, M., & Waters, G. (1990). Effects of reading skill on component spelling skills. *Applied Psycholinguistics, 11,* 425–437.

Bryant, N. D., Drabin, I. R., & Gettinger, M. (1981). Effects of varying unit size on spelling achievement in learning disabled children. *Journal of Learning Disabilities, 14,* 200–203.

Carlisle, J. F. (1987). The use of morphological knowledge in spelling derived forms by learning-disabled and normal students. *Annals of Dyslexia, 37,* 90–108.

Carreker, S. (1992). *Scientific spelling.* Bellaire, TX: Neuhaus Education Center.

Carreker, S. (1999). Teaching spelling. In J. Birsh (Ed.), *Multisensory teaching of basic language skills* (pp. 217–256). Baltimore: Brookes.

Chomsky, C. (1970). Reading, spelling, and phonology. *Harvard Educational Review, 40,* 287–309.

Clarke-Klein, S., & Hodson, B. W. (1995). A phonologically based analysis of misspellings by third graders with disordered-phonology histories. *Journal of Speech and Hearing Research, 38,* 839–849.

Cunningham, A., & Stanovich, K. (1997). Early reading acquisition and its relation to reading experience and ability 10 years later. *Developmental Psychology, 33,* 934–945.

Ehri, L. C. (1989). The development of spelling knowledge and its role in reading acquisition and reading disability. *Journal of Learning Disabilities, 22,* 349–364.

Ehri, L. C., & Robbins, C. (1992). Beginners need some decoding skill to read words by analogy. *Reading Research Quarterly, 27,* 13–26.

Felton, R. H., & Wood, F. B. (1989). Cognitive deficits in reading disability and attention deficit disorder. *Journal of Learning Disabilities, 1,* 3–13.

Fernald, G. (1943). *Remedial techniques in basic school subjects.* New York: McGraw-Hill.

Fink, R. (1998). Literacy development in successful men and women with dyslexia. *Annals of Dyslexia, 48,* 311–346.

Fischer, F. W., Shankweiler, D., & Liberman, I. Y. (1985). Spelling proficiency and sensitivity to word structure. *Journal of Memory and Language, 24,* 423–441.

Fletcher, J. M., & Lyon, G. R. (1998). Reading: A research-based approach. In W. Evers (Ed.), *What's gone wrong in America's classrooms?* Stanford, CA: Stanford University, Hoover Institution.

Frith, U., & Frith, C. (1983). Relationships between reading and spelling. In J. P. Kavanagh & R. L. Venezky (Eds.), *Orthography, reading, and dyslexia*. Baltimore: University Park Press.

Fry, E., Fountoukidis, D. L., & Polk, J. K. (1985). *The new reading teacher's book of lists*. Englewood Cliffs, NJ: Prentice-Hall.

Ganske, K. (2000a). The developmental spelling analysis: A measure of orthographic knowledge. *Educational Assessment, 6(1),* 41–70.

Ganske, K. (2000b). *Word journeys: Assessment, guided phonics, vocabulary, and spelling*. New York: Guilford.

Gillingham, A., & Stillman, B. W. (1997). *Remedial training for children with specific disability in reading, spelling, and penmanship* (8th ed.). Cambridge, MA: Educators Publishing Service.

Greene, J. (1995). *Language!* Longmont, CO: Sopris West.

Henderson, E. (1990). *Teaching spelling* (2nd ed.). Boston: Houghton Mifflin.

Henry, M. (1993). Morphological structure: Latin and Greek roots and affixes as upper grade code strategies. *Reading and Writing: An Interdisciplinary Journal, 5,* 227–241.

Henry, M. (1999). A short history of the English language. In J. Birsh (Ed.), *Multisensory teaching of basic language skills* (pp. 119–133). Baltimore: Brookes.

Henry, M., & Redding, N. (1996). *Patterns for reading and spelling*. Austin, TX: PRO-ED.

Hoffman, P. R., & Norris, J. A. (1989). On the nature of phonological development: Evidence from normal children's spelling errors. *Journal of Speech and Hearing Research, 32,* 787–794.

Invernizzi, M., & Worthy, M. J. (1989). An orthographic-specific comparison of the spelling errors of learning disabled and normal children across four grade levels of spelling achievement. *Reading Psychology: An International Quarterly, 10,* 173–188.

Jastak, S., & Wilkinson, G. S. (1984). *Wide Range Achievement Test*. Wilmington, DE: Jastak Associates.

Johnson, K., & Bayrd, P. (1983). *Megawords*. Cambridge, MA: Educators Publishing Service.

Kaufman, A. S., & Kaufman, N. L. (1985). *Kaufman Test of Educational Achievement*. Circle Pines, MN: American Guidance Service.

Kent, R. D. (1992). The biology of phonological development. In C. A. Ferguson, L. Menn & C. Stoel-Gammon (Eds.), *Phonological development: Models, research, implications* (pp. 65–90). Timonium, MD: York Press.

Kibel, M., & Miles, T. R. (1994). Phonological errors in the spelling of taught dyslexic children. In C. Hulme & M. Snowling (Eds.), *Reading development and dyslexia*. San Diego: Singular.

Larsen, S. C., Hammill, D. D., & Moats, L. (1999). *Test of Written Spelling–Fourth Edition*. Austin, TX: PRO-ED.

Lennox, C., & Siegel, L. S. (1993). Phonological and orthographic processes in good and poor spellers. In C. Hulme & R. M. Joshi (Eds.), *Reading and spelling development and disorders* (pp. 395–404). Mahwah, NJ: Erlbaum.

Liberman, I. Y., Rubin, H., Duques, S., & Carlisle, J. (1985). Linguistic abilities and spelling proficiency in kindergartners and adult poor spellers. In D. B. Gray & J. F. Kavanaugh (Eds.), *Biobehavioral measures of dyslexia* (pp. 163–176). Parkton, MD: York Press.

Liberman, I. Y., Shankweiler, D., & Liberman, A. M. (1989). The alphabetic principle and learning to read. In D. Shankweiler & I. Y. Liberman (Eds.), *Phonology and reading disability: Solving the reading puzzle* (pp. 1–33). Ann Arbor: University of Michigan Press.

Lindamood, P. C., Bell, N., & Lindamood, P. (1992). Issues in phonological awareness assessment. *Annals of Dyslexia, 42,* 242–259.

Lindamood, P., & Lindamood, P. (1998). *The Lindamood phoneme sequencing program for reading, spelling, and speech.* Austin, TX: PRO-ED.

Lombardino, L. J., Riccio, C., Hynd, G. W., & Pinheiro, S. B. (1997). Linguistic deficits in children with reading disabilities. *American Journal of Speech-Language Pathology, 6,* 71–78.

Lyon, G. R. (1995). Toward a definition of dyslexia. *Annals of Dyslexia, 45,* 3–27.

Lyon, G. R., & Moats, L. C. (1988). Critical issues in the instruction of the learning disabled. *Journal of Consulting and Clinical Psychology, 56,* 830–835.

McDonald, G. W., & Cornwall, A. (1995). The relationship between phonological awareness and reading and spelling achievement eleven years later. *Journal of Learning Disabilities, 28,* 523–527.

Moats, L. C. (1983). A comparison of the spelling errors of older dyslexics and second-grade normal children. *Annals of Dyslexia, 33,* 121–139.

Moats, L. C. (1993). Spelling error analysis: Beyond the phonetic/dysphonetic dichotomy. *Annals of Dyslexia, 43,* 174–185.

Moats, L. C. (1996) Phonological spelling errors in the writing of dyslexic adolescents. *Reading and Writing: An Interdisciplinary Journal, 8,* 105–119.

Moats, L. C. (2000). *Speech to print: A course in language study for teachers of reading.* Baltimore: Brookes.

Moats, L. C., & Lyon, G. R. (1993). Learning disabilities in the United States: Advocacy, science, and the future of the field. *Journal of Learning Disabilities, 26,* 282–294.

Moats, L. C., & Smith, C. (1992). Derivational morphology: Why it should be included in assessment and instruction. *Language, Speech and Hearing Services in the Schools, 23,* 312–319.

Nelson, H. E. (1980). Analysis of spelling errors in normal and dyslexic children. In U. Frith (Ed.), *Cognitive Processes in Spelling.* London: Academic Press.

Nulman, J. H., & Gerber, M. M. (1984). Improving spelling performance by imitating a child's errors. *Journal of Learning Disabilities, 17,* 328–333.

Pennington, B. F., McCabe, L. L., Smith, S. D., Lefly, D. L., Bookman, M. O., Kimberling, W. J., & Lubs, H. A. (1986). Spelling errors in adults with a form of familial dyslexia. *Child Development, 57,* 1001–1013.

Rack, J. P., Snowling, M., & Olson, R. K. (1992). The non-word reading deficit in dyslexia: A review. *Reading Research Quarterly 27,* 28–53.

Read, C. (1986). *Children's creative spelling.* London: Routledge and Kegan Paul.

Reith, H., Axelrod, S., Anderson, R., Hathaway, F., Wood, K., & Fitzgerald, C. (1974). Influence of distributed practice and daily testing on weekly spelling tests. *Journal of Educational Research, 68,* 73–77.

Rohl, M., & Tunmer, W. E. (1988). Phonemic segmentation skill and spelling acquisition. *Applied Psycholinguistics, 9,* 335–350.

Sawyer, D., Wade, S., & Kim, J. (1999). Spelling errors as a window on variations in phonological deficits among students with dyslexia. *Annals of Dyslexia, 49.*

Shankweiler, D., Crain, S., Katz, L., Fowler, A. E., Liberman, A. M., Brady, S. A., Thornton, R., Lundquist, E., Dreyer, L., Fletcher, J. M., Stuebing, K. K., Shaywitz, S. E., & Shaywitz, B. A. (1995). Cognitive profiles of reading-disabled children: Comparison of language skills in phonology, morphology, and syntax. *Psychological Science, 6,* 149–156.

Shankweiler, D., Lundquist, E., Dreyer, L., & Dickinson, C. (1996). Reading and spelling difficulties in high school students: Causes and consequences. *Reading and Writing: An Interdisciplinary Journal, 8,* 267–294.

Snow, C., Burns, S., & Griffin, P. (Eds.). (1998). *Preventing reading difficulties in young children.* Washington, DC: National Academy Press.

Snowling, M. J., Goulandris, N., & Defty, N. (1996). A longitudinal study of reading development in dyslexic children. *Journal of Educational Psychology, 88,* 653–659.

Stanovich, K., & Siegel, L. (1994). Phenotypic performance profiles of children with reading disabilities: A regression-based test of the phonological-core variable-difference model. *Journal of Educational Psychology, 86,* 24–53.

Stage, S. A., & Wagner, R. K. (1992). Development of young children's phonological and orthographic knowledge as revealed by their spellings. *Developmental Psychology, 2,* 287–296.

Stuart, M., & Masterson, J. (1992). Patterns of reading and spelling in 10-year-old children related to rereading and phonological abilities. *Journal of Experimental Child Psychology, 54,* 168–187.

Templeton, S., & Bear, D. (Eds.). (1992). *Development of orthographic knowledge and the foundations of literacy: A memorial Festschrift for Edmund H. Henderson.* Hillsdale, NJ: Erlbaum.

Templeton, S., & Morris, D. (1999). Theory and research into practice: Questions teachers ask about spelling. *Reading Research Quarterly, 34,* 102–112.

Treiman, R. (1993). *Beginning to spell: A study of first grade children.* New York: Oxford.

Treiman, R. (1997). Spelling in normal children and dyslexia. In B. Blachman (Ed.), *Foundations of reading acquisition and dyslexia: Implications for early intervention* (pp. 191–218). Mahwah, NJ: Erlbaum.

Viise, N. M. (1992). *A comparison of child and adult spelling development.* Unpublished doctoral dissertation, University of Virginia, Charlottesville.

Wilson, B. A. (1996). *Wilson language program: Instructor manual.* Millbury, MA: Wilson Language Training.

Worthy, M. J., & Invernizzi, M. (1990). Spelling errors of normal and disabled students on achievement levels one through four: Instructional implications. *Annals of Dyslexia, 40,* 138–151.

Handwriting Disorders

Ann M. Bain

U ntil quite recently, handwriting had been like a neglected stepchild of written language, receiving very little attention when compared to that received by reading disorders, although teachers and parents frequently note that handwriting is a struggle for the student with learning disabilities. In 1989, the University of Washington began a research project on writing disabilities funded by the National Institutes of Health. The University of Maryland joined this endeavor in 1995. This West coast–East coast collaboration has launched some exciting and very promising research into writing disorders in general and handwriting development and disorders in particular, though several factors still interact to make handwriting a difficult area for either research or the development of efficacious remedial practices. First, the tenacious nature of handwriting problems is quite discouraging. Often little progress is observed, with the result that little instructional time may be allocated. Second, teachers and parents may covertly believe that handwriting, more so than reading or math, is under the direct control of the student; the student could "perform better if only more effort were put into the task." The problem becomes one of "laziness" or "lack of motivation" rather than one of a learning disability. Another important problem is the real lack of technically sound testing instruments to measure both skill deficit areas and improvement. In addition, efficacious teaching methods are indeed rare. Finally, teachers who instruct children and adults with handwriting deficits often have had little training in either assessment or teaching. This chapter will explore handwriting deficits because they are vitally important in the development of written language. Although the computer offers technological advances for students with handwriting disorders, there are many situations in and out of school in which a person's knowledge, competency, and attitude will be judged through handwriting. If the adult or child with handwriting difficulty does not get help, written language will invariably suffer. Handwriting should be a tool of written language, not a painful, seemingly endless struggle.

Handwriting Development

Handwriting is a difficult, complex task that is learned over a period of time. Luria (1973) suggested that the process of learning letters initially involves memorizing the individual parts of each letter through an interaction between the muscles and kinesthetic feedback. With continued practice, the process changes, and a letter becomes a single movement, an automatized "kinetic melody." It appears that the letter changes from an exclusive visual–motor behavior to an integrated language and visual–motor behavior. Handwriting is indeed "language by hand" (Berninger & Graham, in press), but to what extent is it the underpinning for all of the other aspects of written language? In pioneer neurodevelopmental studies, Berninger and colleagues have analyzed handwriting samples from 900 girls and boys in Grades 1 through 9, which include copying a passage, composing a narrative, and writing an expository paragraph. The children's writing was evaluated for legibility and automaticity. Legibility was assessed by considering the recognizability of a letter independent of the other letters of a word. Automaticity was assessed by timed handwriting samples. As expected, speed increased with grade level but not in regular increments. Legibility also increased with age to peak at Grade 6. Graham and Weintraub (1996) also reported gender differences in writing. In general, girls showed better legibility and speed than boys.

Graham et al. (1997) have investigated the role of handwriting within the process of composing. Berninger and Graham (in press) have theorized that a writer's ability to compose may be taxed if handwriting is not fully automatized because working memory will be relegated to the mechanical task of producing letters rather than the higher level tasks of planning, composing, and editing. Graham (1997) and Berninger and Graham (in press) found that handwriting automaticity has a sizable relation to compositional quality, stronger even than that of spelling. Berninger and Graham stated that, "The degree to which . . . [handwriting] is automatized, that is legible letters can be produced automatically, affects the degree to which working memory resources can be allocated to the cognitive processes in composing" (p. 10). The importance of handwriting automaticity then can hardly be overestimated.

Handwriting Disorders

A breakdown in the writing process may occur in varying degrees at any point in the learning process. D. Johnson and Myklebust (1967) presented a comprehensive differential diagnosis of handwriting disorders including the following: dysgraphia, reading disabilities, visual memory deficits, and motor disorders. Dysgraphia is a visual–motor apraxia. The student with dysgraphia is unable to copy.

Dysgraphia is a disorder resulting from a disturbance in visual–motor integration. The child with this type of involvement has neither a visual nor a motor defect, but he cannot transduce visual information to the motor system. (p. 199)

Other handwriting disorders are the result of different learning disabilities. Students with reading disorders may have trouble writing because they are unable to read. Still other adults and children may have visual memory deficits so that they have difficulty retaining the visual image of letters and numbers. Some students cannot remember or execute the motor movements needed to form letters, words, and numbers; these students have not developed Luria's (1973) kinetic melody.

Terminology

Johnson and Myklebust (1967) used the term *dysgraphia* very precisely; however, many investigators equate the term *dysgraphia* with any number of handwriting, spelling, or written expression disorders in students with learning disabilities. In this chapter, the term *handwriting disorders* will be used to describe the handwriting deficits in children and adults with learning disabilities. A careful differential diagnosis is necessary to determine the nature of the deficit so that appropriate remediation can be planned.

Assessment of Handwriting Disorders

Little is written about the actual behaviors of the student experiencing handwriting difficulty. In my experience, these students often appear to have four characteristics that appear in contiguity: unconventional grip, fingers very near the pencil point, difficulty in erasing, and trouble with letter alignment. Although even the most superficial examination of both adult and child writers shows a myriad of grips, my experience is that many people with handwriting difficulty use a thumb-wrap grip with the pencil held very near the point. This does not appear to vary as the writer changes from cursive to manuscript or vice versa. When a pencil is inverted, this same grip impedes erasing. The individual often erases incompletely and then partially writes over the original marks, thus decreasing overall legibility even more.

Several handwriting behaviors and skills need to be assessed to afford a comprehensive picture of a student's writing. The student's posture, grip, and handedness should be observed. The written production should then be compared to expectations for a student's grade level. There is no formal instrument that includes near- and far-point copying, manuscript and cursive, or writing from memory and spontaneous writing. The clinician must select formal instruments as well as informal tasks to meet the needs of each student.

Standardized Instruments

The few standardized instruments designed to evaluate handwriting are riddled with serious technical problems (Graham, 1982). The *Ayres Handwriting Scale* (Ayres, 1917) is still the most widely used in clinical evaluations. First published in 1912 and later revised in 1917, it was designed to assess the quality and speed of handwriting. In this timed test, the student is instructed to copy the Gettysburg Address at near point from a paper directly in front of him or her. The number of letters written correctly in 1 minute is determined, and then a raw score obtained and converted into a grade-level equivalent. On the positive side, the *Ayres Handwriting Scale* affords the clinician an opportunity to observe the student's writing of the same sample over a period of time. There is, however, a great deal of subjectivity involved in determining what constitutes a well-formed letter. Moreover, little information is available on the reliability and validity of the *Ayres Handwriting Scale*. Osburn (1953) noted that it was not designed to yield diagnostic information. Consequently, the clinician should not be lulled into attending to the score rather than relying on careful observations based on the student's written production and product.

The Handwriting Scale of the *Test of Written Language* (TOWL) (Hammill & Larsen, 1978) is specially designed for assessing cursive writing. The score is derived from examining the child's writing and comparing it to samples in the manual. There are, however, no stated criteria for these levels, which are scores ranging from 1 to 10. On occasion, the child's handwriting does not appear to match any of the samples. In a pilot study using children with learning disabilities, Graham, Boyer-Shick, and Tippets (1989) found that the Handwriting Scale of the TOWL could be considered valid; however, for reliability, the examiners needed more direct training than what was offered in the TOWL manual. The examiners used neatness as an important criterion, which was not even included on any of the TOWL writing samples. Graham et al. (1989) recommended developing new sets of student writing samples and revising the training procedures for examiners. The newest version of the *Test of Written Language,* the TOWL–3 (Hammill & Larsen, 1996), does not include a handwriting subtest.

Several important points addressing the writer and the task should be considered in the development of more comprehensive handwriting instruments. Part of the instrument should include a restandardization of the *Ayres Handwriting Scale,* or a similar writing passage, to measure rate and fluency of copy tasks with developmental norms. In addition, an instrument including writing a timed alphabet and spontaneous writing would be a welcome addition to the field. The development of a standardized instrument for assessing note-taking skills for the older student is also needed. Graham (1986) cautioned that fundamental differences in the age and gender of writers, as well as the relative degree of difficulty of letter formation, should be taken into account when developing better handwriting instruments.

Informal Instruments

Until valid and reliable tests are available, clinical tools that look at the subskills underlying handwriting and posture are needed (Hammill, 1975; Weiser, 1986). The *Handwriting Survey* (Bain, 1995) is a useful informal clinical instrument for recording and systematically describing the student's performance on various handwriting tasks (see Figure 3.1). A variety of handwriting activities appropriate to the age of the student is selected, and observations of posture, grip, handedness, and paper position are recorded. Having the student write the alphabet, as well as single dictated letters, allows the observer to focus on letter formation. Dictated words, generally gleaned from spelling tests, assess the student's connecting strokes, as well as the integration between handwriting and spelling. Assessing these areas is vital since a student might exhibit handwriting deficits, inaccurate spelling, or a combined deficit. The observer should also be alert to the possibility of a bright student masking spelling errors with ambiguous letter formation. With a little imagination, most of the cursive lowercase alphabet could be rendered by writing several loosely formed letters.

Newland (1932) suggested that *r, a, t,* and *e* are the most difficult to form cursive lowercase letters. A close analysis of cursive writing suggests that inordinate difficulty is also encountered with the formation of *m, n,* and the up-and-over or backward-motion letters requiring closure: *a, c, d, g,* and *q*. In addition, the "flag" letters, *b, o, v,* and *w,* are perennial problems. Graham, Weintraub, and Berninger (1998) found that six lowercase manuscript letters (*q, j, z, u, n,* and *k*) accounted for almost half of the errors made by primary-age students in their study.

The differences in performance among the various writing activities can be instructive, particularly in observing the student's approach to the task. Slowness, for instance, may be the result of laboriously copying one letter at a time and frequently losing one's place. It may also be the result of inattentive behavior, retrieval difficulty, or perhaps it may be first writing, then erasing and rewriting.

Although unstandardized, the *Slingerland Screening Tests for Identifying Children with Specific Language Disability* (Slingerland, 1970) represent a step in the right direction, particularly because of the far-point as well

---

Handwriting Survey

Dates _____

Student _____ Observer _____

Age _____ Grade _____ Handed: ☐ right ☐ left ☐ both ☐ undetermined

Teacher _____

Handwriting should be compared on the following activities to describe skills, and to identify any type of problem, the consistency of any problem, and the extent of any difficulty. Specific identification of problems will lead to a remedial plan.

Compare: 1. Write the lowercase alphabet: ☐ manuscript ☐ cursive ☐ both

2. Write the uppercase alphabet: ☐ manuscript ☐ cursive ☐ both

3. Write single words from dictation

4. Copy at near point

5. Copy at far point

6. Write creatively

7. Take notes

8. Compare class work with writing tasks on this survey

On task:

Pencil grip: Position of anchor hand:

Pencil pressure: Position of paper:

Organization of paper (L/R margins; placement of information; sequence of information)

Letter formation: Word formation:

Letter size: Word size:

Letter slant: Word slant:

Letter alignment: Word alignment:

                                          Word spacing:

Additions: Omissions: Substitutions: Reversals:

Erasures: Speed & Fluency:

Attitude toward handwriting:

Other:

Figure 3.1. *Handwriting Survey,* by A. M. Bain, 1995, unpublished manuscript.

as near-point copy tasks. The *Evaluation Tool of Children's Handwriting* (ETCH) (Amundson, 1995) appears to be in the process of standardization. It offers writing of lower- and uppercase alphabets, an illustrated description of pencil grips, writing of numbers, near- and far-point copy, as well as dictation and sentence composition.

In comparing a student's handwriting on the spelling of dictated words, on near- and far-point copy, or within a composition, a pattern of strengths and weaknesses frequently emerges. Handwriting might break down at the level of the composition, perhaps indicating that the integration of spelling, punctuation, ideation, and sentence generation might be an overwhelming task. And, more to the point, handwriting is not fully automatized. A skill deficit at the copying level might indicate inefficient copying strategies or perhaps visual or kinesthetic memory deficits for letters and letter sequences. Difficulty on a spelling task might additionally suggest a spelling deficit or perhaps inadequate auditory processing.

Rate of writing as well as note-taking skills should especially be evaluated for older students whose academic success in some classes is mainly dependent on the efficiency of these skills. Students evidencing a slow rate, inadequate letter formation, or both will have difficulty succeeding academically. Inadequate organizational skills coupled with inefficient handwriting and slow auditory processing produce a combination that leads to incomprehensible notes that are virtually useless in preparing for exams.

The development of a series of transparent overlays (Helwig, 1976; Jones, Trap, & Cooper, 1977) has the potential for the development of a more standard description of handwriting disorders. Ultimately, transparencies may lead to the development of an efficient, valid, and reliable tool for assessing handwriting. It would be useful to include a series of sketches showing hands gripping writing utensils in various positions. For example, the *SEARCH* test (Silver & Hagin, 1976) and the *Evaluation Tool of Children's Handwriting* (Amundson, 1995) contain a partial set of sketches that illustrate pencil grips. (For a look at different grips, see Figures 3.2 and 3.5, which appear later in this chapter.)

Remediation of Handwriting Disorders

Handwriting Materials

Most adult writers are partial to specific pens and pencils ("Inexpensive Pens," 1983), yet developmental handwriting programs are often quite rigid in requiring what paper, pencils, and pens are used in each elementary grade. Surprisingly, the handwriting materials required are based ostensibly on tradition rather than research. Specifications for the materials used in developmental

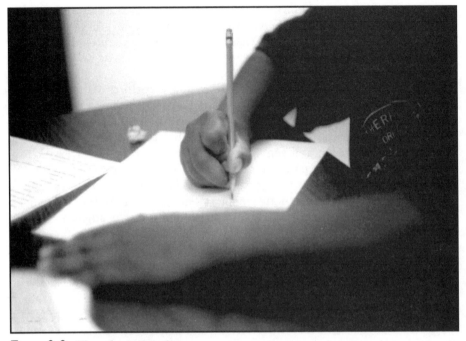

Figure 3.2. Thumb-wrap grip.

programs, such as the type and diameter of writing instruments, as well as the exact amount of space between lines on a paper, are not well documented (Coles & Goodman, 1980; Graham, 1992; Graham & Weintraub, 1996). In individualized remedial programs for students with handwriting deficits, writing materials may even be more important. What types of pencil, pen, and paper are most appropriate? Older students are often unwilling to use the fat, round pencils and wide-ruled paper because these materials are associated with earlier grades. Moreover, the round pencils do not provide useful cues in the development of conventional, comfortable handwriting grips. Many teachers of students with learning disabilities encourage the use of pencil grippers; however, in my experience, the triangular grippers seem to frustrate students, who end up manipulating their hands to work around the gripper or reverting to unconventional hand positions as soon as the grips are removed from the pencil. Still, because the softness of the gripper is comfortable, pencil grippers may be useful for the writer who tends to exert too much pressure on the pencil. It is unclear whether blackboard writing helps the student learn and review letter formation for efficient writing on paper. To varying degrees, many clinicians use the blackboard to teach letter formation, but the transition from a vertical to a horizontal plane may be difficult for some students with learning disabilities. Other students may find that large-muscle exercises done on the board do not prepare them for using the smaller hand muscles required for writing on paper. In planning remedial exercises, the clinician needs to consider the difficulties that students with learning disabilities experience when attempting to generalize and transfer information.

Generally, experimentation with a range of paper, pens, and pencils is most helpful. The student and the therapist can systematically try various materials until maximum comfort is achieved and optimal writing is being produced. Dated samples of the student's work coupled with careful observations are necessary to discover which combination works well for each person.

Remedial Methods

Johnson and Myklebust (1967) presented a comprehensive task-analysis model for the development of a treatment plan, which is necessary when dealing with children and adults with unique learning styles. Graham and Miller (1980) separated and summarized several basic elements used to teach letter formation (see Table 3.1). Modeling is the first step in teaching the student smooth letter production from beginning to end of letter production while describing the critical letter attributes. Physical prompts and cues help the learner to focus on the most critical dimensions of letter formation while tracing allows him or her to practice combining discrete elements into a harmonious whole. Copying helps with a beginning level of automaticity

Table 3.1
Summary of Several Basic Elements Used To Teach Letter Formation

Modeling

Noting critical attributes

Physical prompts and cues

Tracing

Copying

Self-verbalizing

Writing from memory

Repetition

Self-correction and feedback

Note. Adapted from "Handwriting Research and Practice: A Unified Approach," by S. Graham and L. Miller, 1980, *Focus on Exceptional Children, 13*(2), pp. 1–6.

while self-verbalizations probably replace the initial teacher cues. Repetition, self-correction, and feedback, of course, lead to mastery so that higher-level skills can receive the focus of the student's attention.

Remedial methods for handwriting disorders are primarily based on clinical observation. Programs that appear to be most comprehensive because of the number of systematic steps used in teaching cursive letter formation include those by Gillingham and Stillman (1997) and Fernald (1943).

Gillingham and Stillman

1. The teacher models a large letter on the blackboard, writing and saying the letter name.

2. The student traces the letter while saying the name. (The letter sound is sometimes included at the beginning levels of reading.) This tracing stage continues until the student is secure with the letter formation and name.

3. The student copies the letter while saying the name.

4. The student writes the letter from memory while saying the letter name.

Fernald

1. The teacher models the word saying each syllable as naturally as possible, and writing in slightly enlarged letters in crayon on paper.

2. The student traces the word while saying the name of each syllable until he or she is comfortable with the letter formation, directionality, and sequence of syllables.

3. The student then writes the word from memory, usually three times.

Tutors using these Visual, Auditory, Kinesthetic, Tactile (VAKT) approaches will frequently reinforce letter learning by tracing a letter with crayons and magic markers. Sandboxes and saltboxes are also useful for these multisensory experiences in writing. The teacher, with the students, can even use pudding for letter-writing practice. Shaving cream, or other mediums like finger paints, can also be used for writing individual letters and developing connecting strokes. To be efficient writers, children and adults will need a great deal of appropriate practice and systematic review.

A welcome addition to the growing body of literature on remediation is the work of Berninger et al. (1997) and Berninger and Graham (in press). Through meticulous study they have found that providing practice for children by pairing the letter name with the letter formation is an important retrieval cue. They also found that "distributed practice," writing a letter a few times, was more effective than "massed practice," writing rows of the same letter several times. They also found that handwriting practice that provided numbered strokes was more effective than teaching children how to talk their way through the letter strokes.

Readiness Activities

Since writing is primarily a language-based skill, it is unclear whether readiness activities such as drawing and tracing shapes or coloring within lines are effective beyond a kindergarten to a beginning first-grade level. Haworth (1971), Helms (1970), Kepart (1973), Kimmel (1970), and Ramming (1970) all stressed the overall importance of readiness activities. Similarly, Madison (1970) developed a kinesthetic technique with initial writing activities highlighting tracing and copying done in finger paints.

Cues and Prompts

Many handwriting techniques use some sort of physical cue or prompt to help the students with memory and directionality as well as with smoothness of production. Kaliski and Iohga (1970) and Wright (1966) developed music programs for cursive writing. Generally, cursive letters are first grouped according to two-beat (*e, l, c*), three-beat (*t, n, o*), and four-beat (*w, f, g*) letters and then put to music with strong regular beats, such as "The Mexican Hat Dance" and "The Skater's Waltz." A unique program (Dubrow, 1968) that helps students visualize letters uses a technique for teaching lower- and uppercase cursive letters. Each letter is superimposed on the face of a clock and described according to its position. Visualize, for example, Dubrow's analysis of lowercase *i*:

1. Begin at 7 o'clock; swing up toward center.

2. Swing down to 6 and around to 5.

3. Make the dot above the center.

Dotted letters are another kind of prompt widely used with learners of all ages. Powers and Kaminsky (1988) have included a simplified alphabet, dotted letters, and highly structured paper to help students begin to visualize letter proportions.

Butcher (1984) suggested using long straws, feathers, or thin sticks tied to pencils during writing drills to help students become conscious of the position of their pencils during the writing process.

Verbal Cues

Verbal explanations featuring critical details characterize many newer programs, but the research presents mixed results, suggesting that some students with learning disabilities will do well, but others will become confused (Berninger et al., 1997). *The Johnson Handwriting Program,* Level 3 and Ungraded (Johnson, 1977), focuses on critical attributes through a systematic analysis of cursive letters by dissecting and labeling various "control strokes." Verbal explanations for required handwriting motions are advocated by Kirk (1978) and Sovik (1976); however, Robins, Armel, and O'Leary (1975) felt that verbal cues were very difficult for children in kindergarten. Another single case study (Kosiewicz, Hallahan, Lloyd, & Graves, 1982) noted that self-instruction was a very effective strategy for a 9-year-old boy with a learning disability. In a clinical study of 3 children with learning disabilities, Graham (1983) felt that self-verbalizations were difficult either because the verbal cues taught to the children were complex or because the verbalizations actually interfered with the letter-writing tasks. The number of teaching sessions, he felt, may also have been too limited. The point is that children and adults with good oral language skills may do well with self-verbalizations in letter learning, but great care should be taken to assess the difficulty of the script as well as the individual's ongoing progress. Associating the letter name with the grapheme might be the most useful verbal cue (Berninger & Graham, in press).

Self-Evaluation

Nonverbal techniques may be markedly better for some writers who do not have good oral sequential language. A single-subject study (Kosiewicz, Hallahan, & Lloyd, 1981) reviewed basic writing rules, such as staying on the line and proportioning letters, with an 11-year-old child with a learning disability and found an improvement in the child's copying skills. The child was also taught a second strategy that focused on identifying correct letter formation. After the child had copied a paragraph, he was asked to go back and circle correctly formed letters without verbalizations.

Another interesting idea involves the use of transparencies for helping students evaluate their own letter formation (Helwig, 1976; Jones et al., 1977). This intriguing concept may prove invaluable for developing remedial procedures for those students who do not respond well to verbal mediation strategies.

These techniques are, of course, often combined to formulate different remedial programs and strategies. The question is which combination to use for which learner. A secondary issue is ongoing assessment and evaluation so that the child or adult does not stagnate at any level but also is not pushed to the point of frustration. Care should be taken that the type of reinforcement is appropriate to the age and needs of the student. Although many questions remain unanswered in the area of handwriting, clinicians frequently employ several of these approaches to remediation, which suggests some validity to each technique.

Additional Skills

Generally, the person with writing deficits does not acquire handwriting skills incidentally or transfer them spontaneously. Clinicians will need to plan precise instruction on copying at near point and far point. Students will also need to learn to incorporate newly learned handwriting skills into spontaneous written language through a great deal of focused practice. Berninger et al. (1997) structured their remediation to include writing a composition at the end of each short, direct handwriting practice to help children transfer newly learned skills into writing compositions. Older students will also need explicit instruction in note taking skills. Teachers can provide a shell of an outline with sufficient space allotted for student notes. This kind of overall structure is especially useful for the novice note-taker.

Cursive or Manuscript

Although many specialists have advocated the use of cursive writing for students with learning disabilities (Fernald, 1943; Gillingham & Stillman, 1960; Mullins, Joseph, Turner, Zawadyski, & Saltzman, 1972), little solid data actually support this notion (Peck & Fairchild, 1980) for the student with handwriting problems. In fact, sometimes manuscript appears to be easier and more legible for children with severe handwriting problems. In the large study of 900 children in Grades 1 through 9 (Graham et al., 1998, as described in Berninger & Graham, in press), there was an unexpected twist to the manuscript–cursive debate. There were no statistically significant differences between manuscript and cursive writing in either legibility or speed. Interestingly enough, however, students who mixed manuscript and cursive letters showed as legible, if not more legible, writing than either manuscript or cursive writing alone. The students who used mixed manuscript–cursive writing also tended to write faster than the students who used solely either manuscript or cursive letters. It may prove to be almost as important as to how the cursive or manuscript program is actually individualized for the child with handwriting problems as to whether cursive or manuscript is actually chosen as the actual handwriting program (Graham, in press). The debate over cursive and manuscript will continue until there is an added research base describing students with dysgraphia. Careful clinical studies should produce a profile of the student most likely to succeed with manuscript or cursive rather than attempt to generalize to all students with learning disabilities.

Compensatory Devices

For students with persistent handwriting difficulties, the development of compensatory strategies may be vital for academic success as well as for a positive self-image. Oral testing or objective tests can be substituted for written exams. Although somewhat time-consuming for an entire test, the tape recorder can be used by the student in lieu of lengthy written essays. In addition, the tape recorder can be an invaluable backup support for the student who is an inefficient note-taker because of handwriting or auditory processing deficits. Teachers can greatly assist these students by providing copies of notes from students who are expert note-takers. Teachers can also provide keyword notes for the student to fill in during a class presentation. Most important, teachers need to model how to expand these notes and to provide sufficient practice so that students will have valuable tools for studying. Still another alternative is to teach the student typing skills (Duffy, 1974; King, 1985; Nash & Geyer, 1983) for a word processor (Daiute, 1985). It should be noted, however, that neither does the student develop proficiency magically nor does keyboarding totally eliminate the need for handwriting. With the many technological advances occurring almost daily, such as the laptop computer, the possibilities for compensatory devices seem almost limitless. However, three points should be kept in mind. First, whatever the compensatory device, both direct instruction and daily supervised practice time will be needed for mastery; word processing or efficient use of a tape recorder are not overnight projects. Second, compensatory devices are not substitutes for a carefully designed remedial handwriting program. Third, since students who have handwriting disorders may have apraxia, keyboarding for them would be quite difficult. On the other hand, students with handwriting disorders may also evidence oral language disorders, suggesting that a tape recorder would not be a useful compensatory device. The point is that the strengths and deficits of each student must be analyzed carefully in planning remedial and compensatory programs.

 David

David is an 11-year, 11-month-old, seventh-grader referred for psychoeducational testing because of difficulty with written language. He had received a psychological evaluation the year before, but his parents were concerned because David was making little academic progress and becoming increasingly more discouraged with his schoolwork. There is a positive paternal family history of both handwriting and spelling disorders. (See Table 3.2 for David's psychoeducational testing results.)

Test Behavior

David stated that he is particularly ashamed of his poor handwriting and finds that he limits written expression to a minimum. He noted that most school subjects were just "OK," although he was slightly more enthusiastic about science, in which competency was judged through experiments and occasional oral reports.

Handwriting

Although David used a conventional right-hand grip, his fingers were positioned almost on the tip of the pencil. Pressure appeared adequate. The position of the left hand was variable; sometimes David held the paper, but at other times he held his head, letting the paper slide as he wrote. When the left hand anchored the paper, legibility was slightly improved.

For this evaluation David chose manuscript, which he uses for all writing situations (see Figure 3.3). In general his writing appeared illegible, with letter malformations being the single most important factor. Most difficulty was noted with letters requiring closure and curvature, such as *a, o, r, d,* and *f.* Inconsistent letter formation also contributed to decreased legibility. Letter and word spacing were somewhat variable but not a major area of concern. Handwriting was slightly better on isolated letters. As the length of writing tasks increased, legibility decreased.

Cursive letter formation was slow and halting because of David's lack of familiarity with many letters and because of problems with directionality. Number formation was also inadequate; moreover, David had difficulty aligning numbers in columns. He also tended to write over, rather than erase completely. These handwriting problems accounted for most of his math errors observed during the evaluation.

Written Language

David wrote a very interesting story in response to the TOWL (see Figures 3.3, handwritten, and 3.4, typed). The story was elaborate, creative, and well organized. When highly structured picture cues were not presented, however, David experienced difficulty in organizing his written work. He did not evidence any apparent prewriting or editing strategies.

Proofreading for Mechanics

David was able to proofread for grammar and punctuation on structured tasks but could not apply this skill to his own work.

Table 3.2
David's Psychoeducational Testing Results

Previously Administered Tests:

WISC–R: VIQ: 141   PIQ: 124   FSIQ: 137 (subtests unavailable)

Test of Written Language: Standard Score 103 (subtests unavailable)

Selected Tests of Current Evaluation	Grade Equivalent	Percentile
Wide Range Achievement Test–3 (Wilkinson, 1993)		
Spelling (dictated)	5.7	37
Arithmetic (computation)	10.5	99
Woodcock Reading Mastery Tests–Revised (Woodcock, 1987)		
Letter Identification (no errors)		
Word Identification	6.2	38
Word Attack	5.1	34
Word Comprehension	12.9	91
Passage Comprehension	9.2	64
Total Reading	8.2	62
Gray Oral Reading Tests–3 (Wiederholt & Bryant, 1992)	6.7	
Test of Written Language–3 (Hammill & Larsen, 1996)		
Vocabulary		84
Thematic Maturity		91
Word Usage		84
Style		91

Diagnostic Inventory–Level II (Informal)	Percent Correct
Spelling Regular Words	40%
Doubling Rule	60%
Drop the *e* Rule	80%
/ŏŏ/ and /ōō/	100%
oi and *oy*	100%
/ā/	100%
/ī/	100%
/ō/	40%
–*dge* and –*ge*	100%
–*ck* and –*k*	80%

Note. WISC–R = *Wechsler Intelligence Scale for Children–Revised* (Wechsler, 1974); VIQ = Verbal IQ; PIQ = Performance IQ; FSIQ = Full Scale IQ.

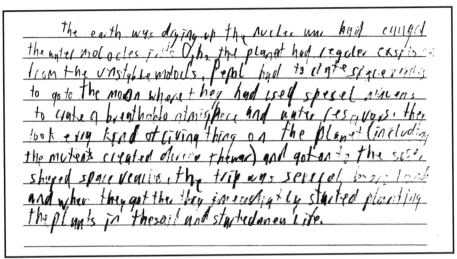

Figure 3.3. David's response to the *Test of Written Language*.

Grade 7 TOWL

The earth was drying up the cucler war and chnged the water molocles into O_1h_2 the planet had reguler exsplosons from the unstable molocls. Peopl had to crnte {create} space veacles to go to the moon where they had used spesel (special) macens {machines} to crate {create} a breathable atmispere and water resavors. they took evry kind of living thing on the planet (including the mutents {mutants} created during the war) and got on to the suser {saucer} haped veacles. the trip ans {was?} hoers long and when they got ther they imeadiatey started planting the plants in the soil and started a new life.

Figure 3.4. David's response to the *Test of Written Language* with handwriting factored out.

Diagnostic Impressions

David appears to be a child who is both gifted and learning disabled, with specific deficits in handwriting, spelling, and written language.

Recommendations

For bright students like David who have specific learning disabilities, recommendations must be for the immediate problems as well as for the student's future aspirations. Both remediation and compensation must be considered—not one or the other. Students like David can pursue their dreams of higher education if they do not get discouraged in the middle school and high school years.

1. In spelling, activities discussed in Chapter 2 of this book would be appropriate.

2. In the area of handwriting, several techniques would be useful:

   A. David and his tutor will need to decide to use either cursive or on manuscript.

   B. The importance of posture, position of the anchor hand, and pencil grip should be emphasized.

   C. Either *The Johnson Handwriting Program* (1977), Write Right—or Left program (Hagin, 1983), or *Handwriting: A Fresh Start* (Powers & Kaminsky, 1988) should be explored since David responded well to analyzing letter strokes and verbal cues during this evaluation. Letter formation in these programs is simplified.

   D. David and his tutor and teachers should decide on the writing standard acceptable for school assignments (which at this point should be kept to a minimum). As his writing begins to improve, the standard of quality, as well as length of the handwriting assignments, should reflect his growth.

3. David will also need some compensatory strategies because of his severe handwriting disorder.

   A. Oral reports should be substituted for written ones. This would include the possibility of using a tape recorder.

   B. He may have a "buddy" to copy board assignments, but David would need to reciprocate in an area of strength, such as math.

   C. Rather than recopying math problems or spelling exercises, David will need workbooks in which he can write.

   D. David would greatly benefit from learning to use the computer. Keyboarding skills should be taught and practiced on a daily basis. Moreover, he may improve his written language through strategies suggested in Chapter 5 of this book.

4. In written expression, David would benefit specifically from learning strategies from the Process Approach to Writing discussed in Chapter 6 of this book.

Mort

Mort is an 11-year, 1-month-old male who was referred for a comprehensive evaluation because of a sudden drop in school grades, deteriorating handwriting, and increased behavior problems at home.

Pediatric Evaluation

Past medical history is significant for meningitis at age 5 requiring a 12-day hospitalization and antibiotics. In the second grade Mort was noted to have had an eye tic without refractive error. He had developed increasing tics more recently, which included shoulder shrugging, head nodding with vocalization, and barking noises. In addition, he has some throat-clearing vocalizations and abdominal contractions. He has had no echolalia or coprolalia. The results of electroencephalography and magnetic resonance imaging were within normal limits.

Psychoeducational Evaluation: Test Behavior

Mort is planning to enter the sixth grade in September. During a recent evaluation (see results in Table 3.3), Mort appeared as a cooperative and friendly youngster with an excellent background of experience and age-appropriate attention to task. Mort evidenced head nodding with vocalizations during the evaluation. He stated that he is quite concerned about his difficulty in school, particularly in math and handwriting.

Handwriting

Mort used his right hand with an unconventional grip (see Figure 3.5). He held his thumb tucked underneath his index finger and appeared to exert excessive pressure while writing. The eraser of the pencil often pointed outward over his knuckles. Mort held his left hand on the top of the paper to anchor it. For this evaluation he chose cursive writing, which is required in his school program. He evidenced difficulty with the up-and-over letters, such as *c*, *o*, and *a*. He also had trouble with *y*, *z*, *u*, *v*, and *s*. Connecting strokes, most notably with the flag letters (*b*, *o*, *w*, and *v*), were also problematic. Mort also tended to write over rather than erase, thus decreasing overall legibility. Spacing and slant appeared satisfactory, but he had difficulty estimating the right paper margin. An analysis of math errors indicated that Mort frequently had difficulty solely with number alignment.

Table 3.3

Selected Test Results for Mort

WISC–R Verbal IQ: 107		Performance IQ: 106	Full Scale IQ: 107
Information	12	Picture Completion	11
Similarities	10	Picture Arrangement	12
Arithmetic	9	Block Design	13
Vocabulary	11	Object Assembly	9
Comprehension	14	Coding	10

	Standard Score	Percentile	Grade Equivalent
Wide Range Achievement Test–3 (Wilkinson, 1993)			
Spelling (dictated)	118	88	
Test of Written Language–3 (Hammill & Larsen, 1996)			
Vocabulary	9	37	
Thematic Maturity	10	50	
Woodcock–Johnson Psycho-Educational Battery–R (Woodcock & Johnson, 1989)			
Math Cluster			4.8
Calculations			
Applied Problems			
Handwriting Survey (informal)			

Note. WISC–R = *Wechsler Intelligence Scale for Children–Revised* (Wechsler, 1974).

Written Expression

Mort wrote a clever, humorous response to the TOWL (see Figure 3.6). Although he did not demonstrate any obvious prewriting skills, the beginning and middle of his story were well planned; however, a definite ending was not included. Mort's school writing assignments that do not include such a structured writing prompt show more writing organizational deficits.

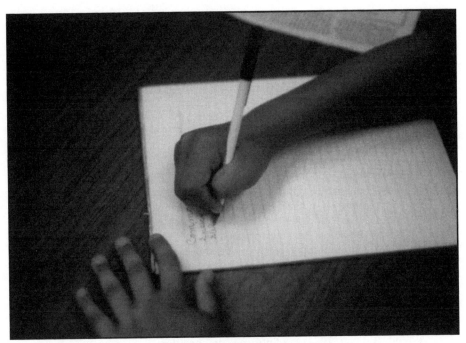

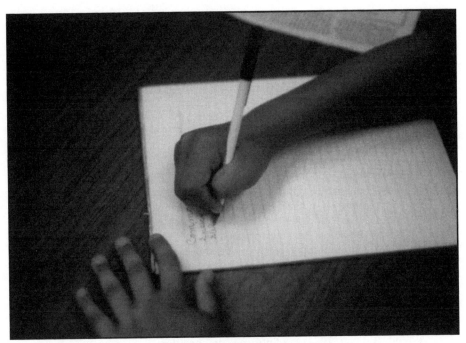

Figure 3.5. Mort's unconventional pencil grip.

Figure 3.6. Mort's response to the *Test of Written Language*.

Diagnostic Impressions

1. Rule out Tourette's syndrome

2. Specific learning disability in handwriting

Recommendations

1. Mort is referred to the Tourette's clinic for an evaluation.

2. Several handwriting techniques would be useful.

   A. Mort would probably do better with manuscript writing because it is easier to control. With the cooperation of his school as well as with his permission, a trial, from September through Thanksgiving, using manuscript could be made with dated samples of his work kept in a folder. Short periods of structured practice on a daily basis are suggested. In November, both cursive and manuscript writing should be reevaluated on the basis of legibility, ease of writing, and rate.

   B. Mort should be taught how to estimate space to the right margin. Of course, he should also be given paper with a visible margin.

   C. He should be given short exercises with a straw attached to his pencil (Butcher, 1984) to reinforce pencil position.

   D. Graph paper should be provided for math problems because of his significant difficulty aligning numbers.

   E. Keyboarding should be taught at school so that the computer can become a useful tool for him. Daily practice periods are also necessary.

References

Amundson, S. J. (1995). *Evaluation Tool of Children's Handwriting*. Homer, AK: O.T. KIDS.

Ayres, L. P. (1917). *Ayres Scale for Measuring Handwriting*. Princeton, NJ: Educational Testing Service.

Bain, A. M. (1995). *Handwriting survey*. Unpublished manuscript.

Berninger, V., & Graham, S. (in press). Language by hand: A synthesis of a decade of research in handwriting. *Handwriting Review*.

Berninger, V., Vaughan, K., Abbott, R., Abbott, S., Rogan, L., & Reed, E. (1997). Treatment of handwriting problems in beginning writers: Transfer from handwriting to composition. *Journal of Educational Psychology, 89*(4), 652–666.

Butcher, E. (1984, October). *Teaching handwriting to LD students*. Paper presented at the conference of the Metropolitan Association of Children with Learning Disabilities, Towson, MD.

Coles, R. E., & Goodman, Y. (1980). Do we really need those oversized pencils to write with? *Theory into Practice, 19*(3), 194–196.

Daiute, C. (1985). *Writing & computers*. Reading, MA: Addison-Wesley.

Dubrow, H. (1968). *Learning to write* (Book 2). Cambridge, MA: Educators Publishing Service.

Duffy, J. (1974). *Type it*. Cambridge, MA: Educators Publishing Service.

Fernald, G. (1943). *Remedial techniques in basic school subjects*. New York: McGraw-Hill.

Gillingham, A., & Stillman, B. W. (1960). *Remedial training for children with specific disability in reading, spelling, and penmanship*. Cambridge, MA: Educators Publishing Service.

Gillingham, A., & Stillman, B. (1997). *The Gillingham manual*. Cambridge, MA: Educators Publishing Service.

Graham, S. (1982). Measurement of handwriting skills: A critical review. *Diagnostique, 8*, 32–42.

Graham, S. (1983). The effect of self-instructional procedures on LD students' handwriting performance. *Learning Disability Quarterly, 6*, 231–234.

Graham, S. (1986). The reliability, validity, and utility of three handwriting measurement procedures. *Journal of Educational Research, 79*(6), 373–380.

Graham, S. (1992). Issues in handwriting instruction. *Focus on Exceptional Children, 25*(2), 1–14.

Graham, S. (1997). Executive control in the revising of students with learning and writing difficulties. *Journal of Educational Psychology, 89*, 223–234.

Graham, S. (in press). Handwriting and spelling instruction for students with learning disabilities: A review. *Learning Disabilities Quarterly*.

Graham, S., Berninger, V., Abbott, R., Abbott, S., & Whitaker, D. (1997). Role of mechanics in composing of elementary school students: A new methodological approach. *Journal of Educational Psychology, 89*, 170–182.

Graham, S., Boyer-Shick, K., & Tippets, E. (1989). The validity of the handwriting scale from the *Test of Written Language*. *Journal of Educational Research, 82*(3), 166–171.

Graham, S., & Miller, L. (1980). Handwriting research and practice: A unified approach. *Focus on Exceptional Children, 13*(2), 1–6.

Graham, S., & Weintraub, N. (1996). A review of handwriting research: Progress and prospects from 1980 to 1994. *Educational Psychology Review, 8*(1), 7–87.

Graham, S., Weintraub, N., & Berninger, V. (1998). The relationship between handwriting style and speed and legibility. *The Journal of Educational Research, 91*(5), 290–296.

Hagin, R. (1983). Write right—or left: A practical approach to handwriting. *Journal of Learning Disabilities, 16*(5), 266–271.

Hammill, D. (1975). Problems in writing. In D. Hammill & N. Bartel (Eds.), *Teaching children with learning and behavior problems* (pp. 149–171). Boston: Allyn & Bacon.

Hammill, D., & Larsen, S. (1978). *Test of Written Language.* Austin, TX: PRO-ED.

Hammill, D. D., & Larsen, S. C. (1996). *Test of Written Language–Third Edition.* Austin, TX: PRO-ED.

Haworth, M. (1971). The effects of rhythmic-motor training and gross-motor training on the reading and handwriting abilities of educable mentally retarded children. *Dissertation Abstracts International, 31*, 3391–A.

Helms, H. B. (1970). Big chalkboard for big movement. In J. Arena (Ed.), *Building handwriting skills in dyslexic children.* San Rafael, CA: Academic Therapy.

Helwig, J. (1976). Measurement of visual-verbal feedback on changes in manuscript letter formation. *Dissertation Abstracts International, 36*, 5196–A.

Inexpensive pens. (1983). *Consumer's Report*, pp. 229–233.

Johnson, D., & Myklebust, H. (1967). *Learning disabilities: Educational principles and practices.* New York: Grune & Stratton.

Johnson, W. T. (1977). *The Johnson Handwriting Program.* Cambridge, MA: Educators Publishing Service.

Jones, J. C., Trap, J., & Cooper, J. (1977). Technical report: Students' self-recording of manuscript letter strokes. *Journal of Applied Behavior Analysis, 10*, 509–514.

Kaliski, L., & Iohga, R. (1970). A musical approach to handwriting. In J. Arena (Ed.), *Building handwriting skills in dyslexic children* (pp. 45–51). San Rafael, CA: Academic Therapy.

Kepart, N. C. (1973). Developmental sequences. In S. Sapir & A. Nitzburg (Eds.), *Children with learning problems.* New York: Brunner/Mazel.

Kimmel, G. M. (1970). Handwriting readiness: Motor-coordinative practices. In J. Arena (Ed.), *Building handwriting skills in dyslexic children* (pp. 101–103). San Rafael, CA: Academic Therapy.

King, D. (1985). *Writing skills for the adolescent.* Cambridge, MA: Educators Publishing Service.

Kirk, U. (1978). Rule-based instruction. A cognitive approach to beginning handwriting instruction. *Dissertation Abstracts International, 39*, 113–A.

Kosiewicz, M., Hallahan, D., & Lloyd., J. (1981). The effects of an LD student's treatment choice on handwriting performance. *Learning Disability Quarterly, 4*(3), 281–286.

Kosiewicz, M., Hallahan, D., Lloyd., & Graves, A. (1982). Effects of self-instruction and self-correction procedures on handwriting performance. *Learning Disability Quarterly, 5*(1), 71–79.

Luria, A. (1973). *The working brain.* London: Penguin Books.

Madison, B. D. (1970). A kinesthetic technique for handwriting development. In J. Arena (Ed.), *Building handwriting skills in dyslexic children* (pp. 17–18). San Rafael, CA: Academic Therapy.

Mullins, J., Joseph, F., Turner, C., Zawadyski, R., & Saltzman, L. (1972). A handwriting model for children with learning disabilities. *Journal of Learning Disabilities, 5*, 306–311.

Nash, K., & Geyer, C. (1983). *Touch to type.* North Billerica, MA: Curriculum Associates.

Newland, E. (1932). An analytic study of the development of illegibilities in handwriting from the lower grades to adulthood. *Journal of Educational Research, 26*, 249–258.

Osburn, W. (1953). Handwriting. In O. Buros (Ed.), *Fourth mental measurements yearbook*. Highland Park, NJ: Gryphon Press.

Peck, M., & Fairchild, S. H. (1980). Another decade of research in handwriting: Progress and prospect in the 1970s. *Journal of Educational Research, 73*(5), 283–289.

Powers, R., & Kaminsky, S. (1988). *Handwriting: A fresh start*. North Billerica, MA: Curriculum Associates.

Ramming, J. (1970). Using the chalkboard to overcome handwriting difficulties. In J. Arena (Ed.), *Building handwriting skills in dyslexic children* (pp. 85–87). San Rafael, CA: Academic Therapy.

Robins, A., Armel, S., & O'Leary, K. (1975). The effects of self-instruction on writing deficiencies. *Behavior Therapy, 6,* 178–187.

Silver, A. A., & Hagin, R. A. (1976). *SEARCH*. New York: Walker Educational Book Corp.

Slingerland, B. (1970). *Slingerland Screening Tests for Identifying Children with Specific Language Disability*. Cambridge, MA: Educators Publishing Service.

Sovik, N. (1976). The effects of different principles of instruction in children's copying performance. *Journal of Experimental Education, 45,* 38–45.

Wechsler, D. (1974). *Wechsler Intelligence Scale for Children–Revised*. San Antonio: Psychological Corporation.

Weiser, D. (1986). Handwriting: Assessment of remediation. *Developmental Disabilities, 9*(3), 1–3.

Wiederholt, J. L., & Bryant, B. R. (1992). *Gray Oral Reading Tests–Third Edition*. Austin, TX: PRO-ED.

Wilkinson, G. S. (1993). *Wide Range Achievement Test–Third Edition*. Wilmington, DE: Wide Range.

Woodcock, R. W. (1987). *Woodcock Reading Mastery Tests–Revised*. Circle Pines, MN: American Guidance Service.

Woodcock, R. W., & Johnson, W. B. (1989). *Woodcock–Johnson Psycho-Educational Battery–Revised*. Itasca, IL: Riverside.

Wright, E. (1966). *Handwriting to music*. Paper presented at the July summer training session of Reading Research Institute, Fryeburg, ME.

Disorders of Written Expression

Noel Gregg and Teresa Hafer

Written expression is a complex form of communication requiring the integration of many different cognitive and linguistic variables. As the demands of literacy increase within our society, the need to better discern the processes that impact on the understanding and production of written text are more a matter of pragmatic necessity than theoretical interest. A mastery of basic written expression skills has become a prerequisite for the majority of jobs graduates of our school systems face today.

Written expression requires that the writer simultaneously deal with a subject, text, and reader; breakdowns in the system may occur for several different reasons. Written expression is certainly dependent on a writer's experiences as well as oral language and reading competencies. The purpose of this chapter is to explore written expression at the sentence and text level and the constraints that can impact a child's, adolescent's, or adult's ability to connect ideas to written text. Other chapters in this book explore spelling and handwriting abilities that also contribute to written expression competence.

History of the Clinical Syndrome

The term *dysgraphia* has historically been applied to disorders of written language without a clear description of the term. The majority of investigations regarding dysgraphia have been based on research specifically focusing only on spelling. The impact of developmental disorders on acquisition of written language at the sentence and text levels has not been the focus of as much research.

Myklebust's (1965) seminal publication of the theory and application of the *Picture Story Language Test* described several processes impacting the ability to generate written discourse. Although the cognitive processes

103

Myklebust (1965) identified as resulting in dysgraphia have been questioned by current research, the contribution of his work in the area of developmental writing disorders should not be underestimated today. Myklebust explored the breakdown of written expression at the word, sentence, and text levels. In addition, he very clearly defined the term dysgraphia from a developmental perspective, differentiating it from ataxia and paralytic disorders. Myklebust used the term dysgraphia to apply only to disorders symbolic in nature. In such cases, he felt a breakdown occurred between the mental image of the word and the motor system. Therefore, Myklebust was one of the first to describe the symbolic nature of dysgraphia. Recently Graham and Weintraub (1996) stressed this same point by concluding that the "production processes involving semantic, syntactic, lexical and phonological factors affect the execution and the production of the motor processes involved in writing" (p. 18).

Myklebust (1965) based his research on a serial hierarchical processing model that has been replaced by theories that propose the concept of neuro-networking. Such theories are based on the premise that networks of neuroanatomical entities are configured by different functional demands so that a given neuroanatomical entity may contribute to different functions (Deuel & Collins, 1984; Getting, 1989). Written expression requires interactions between neural systems; Berninger (1996) referred to this as "crosstalk."

The impact of social context on the development of writing ability has been the focus of much research in the area of written expression. The sociolinguistic model infers that social relationships and culture are the "sources of the mind, the working brain only its organ, and the unique social activity of each subject how it originates" (Blanck, 1990, p. 49). Luria (1981) expressed this same idea in different words: "One must seek the origins of conscious activity and 'categorical' behavior not in the recesses of the human brain or in the depths of the spirit, but in the external conditions of life" (p. 25). Gregg (1995) stressed the need for the use of an integrated model of written expression, one that combines both a neuropsychological and a sociolinguistic framework.

Cause or Constraint

Identifying the source of breakdowns in written expression requires one to consider two important concepts, causality and constraints. Causality infers that one can identify the cause(s) of specific writing disorders. Current cognitive processes that researchers are investigating as possibly impacting written expression include executive functions (Graham, 1997), working memory (Berninger, 1999; McCutchen, 1996), and phonology and orthography (Berninger, 1999; Graham, 1999; Graham & Weintraub, 1996). Since sufficient research has not yet been conducted to allow us to identify the specific cause(s) for writing disorders, the term *constraints* is more helpful in work-ing with individuals with developmental writing problems. Constraints are barriers that make writing difficult but do not constitute the single cause of breakdowns in communication. Examples of constraints could be the lack of any of the following: instruction, oral language abilities, cognitive abilities, neurodevelopment, or motivation. "Learning is 'caused' by the net effect of these various constraints, the influence of which may vary depending upon what is happening at the other levels of constraint" (Berninger, 1996, p. 25).

Process Approach to Writing

Vygotsky (1978) described writing as an active, social, problem-solving pro-cess that should be taught in a meaningful context. The work of Brown and Palinscar (1988) on reciprocal teaching provides an excellent example of how semiotic mediated interpsychological functioning (between self and others) in the classroom can be transformed to intrapsychological functioning (inner dialogue) by applying Vygotskian principles. During the last several years, the process approach to the understanding and teaching of writing as a problem-solving activity has been explored by several researchers. As Wertsch (1998) stated, the importance is not to focus on only the individual psychological aspect of learning. "The point is to think of this as a moment of action rather than as a separate process or entity that exists some how in solution" (p. 23).

A cognitive model of the writing process based on protocol analysis of adult writers "thinking aloud" as they composed was proposed by Hayes and Flower (1980). Out of this research, Hayes and Flower identified three pro-cesses—planning, translating, and reviewing—that writers use in translat-ing ideas into written symbols. A major contribution of the Hayes and Flower model was the observation that the writing process is recursive, meaning that planning, translating, and reviewing are processes used by a writer not sequentially but interactively throughout the writing process.

Berninger et al. (1992) elaborated on the translation stage of the Hayes and Flower (1980) process model of writing. They felt that Hayes and Flower did not distinguish adequately between idea generation and text generation. Therefore, they further broke down the translation process from the Hayes and Flower model into text generation and transcription. According to Berninger (1996), text generation is the "transforming of ideas into language in working memory" and "transcription is the translating of those language representations in working memory into written symbols on the printed page" (p. 133). Transcription is more heavily loaded at the earlier stages of writing while text generation plays a more dominant role as linguistic skills develop. Both processes develop at different rates across writers.

The process approach offers an advantage to those working with writers demonstrating developmental writing disorders. It is based on a problem-solving or cognitive model of writing that values authentic reasons for writing while encouraging an ongoing dialogue between instructor and writer (Graham, Harris, McArthur, & Schwartz, 1991; Hallenbeck, 1996). However, criticism of the process approach has centered on its lack of guidelines for skill development and evaluation (Michaels & O'Connor, 1990).

Responding to the need for skill development and evaluation to be incorporated into a process approach to writing, Englert (1990) introduced the Cognitive Strategy in Writing (CSIW) methodology for teaching written expression. Such an approach combines the process writing theory with an emphasis on text structure and cognitive writing strategies (Englert & Palincsar, 1991). Englert (1990, 1992) based the CSIW approach on the social constructivist framework of Vygotsky (1978). The CSIW model presents writing as a holistic activity learned best from teachers modeling the thinking and inner talk underlying the writing process (Hallenbeck, 1996). Writing is seen as a social activity best learned in authentic situations.

Identifying Developmental Expressive Formulation Writing Disorders

A single assessment tool should never be the sole means of determining whether an individual exhibits a written language disorder. Luria (1980) described a series of tasks designed to analyze the "state of the various elementary components and levels of writing" (p. 537) that can guide professionals developing assessment tools in the area of written expression. Luria advocated always including copy, dictation, and spontaneous tasks when evaluating written expression at the word, sentence, or text level.

Copying

Luria (1980) suggested asking the student being evaluated to copy individual letters, single words, isolated sentences, and paragraphs, depending on his or her age. Spelling, syntax, and organizational deficits can be noted as the demands of the task increase. Luria also recommended varying the type of script (size, density, and type) to assess specific motor and visual processing abilities. The copying of nonsense words (Roeltgen, 1985) is also valuable since it is more difficult to transcribe figures with no apparent symbolic meaning and will better measure true phonological and orthographic competencies. Varying the time interval between the presentation of the letter, word, or sentence and the moment when the individual is allowed to reproduce the information was suggested by Luria (1980) as a means to evaluate how long a student can mentally hold images before transcribing them onto paper. Monitoring the strategies an individual uses (e.g., speaking out loud, tracing), as well as the amount of time necessary to complete the task, provides information critical to drawing conclusions regarding the presence of a disorder versus a learning style or instructional difference.

Dictation

The ability to complete a dictation task requires the individual to integrate auditory, visual, and motor skills in an automatic manner. Therefore, dictation tasks should include the writing of letters, syllables, and sentences. In order to distinguish between possible linguistic or motor breakdowns, the examiner might use anagrams (blocks with single letters written on them) to modify the response mode.

Spontaneous Writing

A spontaneous writing sample would require the individual to write either a sentence, a paragraph, or a story on a familiar topic. Many researchers have indicated that such a task requires extensive integration of several cognitive and linguistic processes (Cromer, 1980; Gregg, 1989; Luria, 1980; Roeltgen, 1985). The complexity of the stimuli (sentence starter, picture, or topic) will also significantly influence the student's performance. It is imperative that the examiner choose types of stimuli that will elicit the best performances from the student.

Written Syntax

A dearth of information exists regarding the types of syntactical error patterns indicative of individuals with developmental writing disorders, as well as appropriate instruments useful in documenting such errors. An understanding of the constraints impacting syntax development would help the refinement of more appropriate identification and instructional strategies. As Shaughnessy (1977) illustrated, error-laden work should be viewed in light of its intentional structures as evidence of systematic, rule-governed behavior.

Written syntax problems often reflect underlying oral language (receptive or expressive) syntax disorders. Therefore, a diagnostician should compare the oral language to the written language of any student where concern for written syntax is under investigation. Figures 4.1 and 4.2 provide evaluation results and oral and written samples from Chip, a freshman in college. The

---

Age: 22 years old

School: College Freshman

Evaluation Results:

Results of a thorough psychological evaluation indicated that Chip demonstrated significant deficits in working memory, phonological awareness, speed of processing, and motor tasks. He found it difficult to pronounce multisyllabic words, resulting in hesitations, omissions, and dysfluency in oral language (see language sample below). Although Chip enjoyed listening to conversations on topics requiring abstract reasoning due to his superior reasoning and thinking skills, he found it difficult to express verbally what he was thinking. His written language was impaired by poor spelling, word substitutions, word omissions, and morphological omissions (see written language sample, Figure 4.2). Significant word finding and expressive syntax problems were apparent during any tasks requiring Chip to respond orally.

Chip's strengths were noted in verbal and nonverbal reasoning. Particular strengths were noted on measures of visual creativity and nonverbal problem solving. In his written expression, he demonstrated strengths in ideation, sense of audience, and text structure. On measures of listening comprehension and reading comprehension, he performed above average.

Oral Language Sample:

WHERE WILL I BE NOW – IN FIFTEEN YEARS NOW. THAT'S THE QUESTION – OF THIS CONSERVATION. FIFTEEN YEARS FROM NOW I WILL LIKE TO BE I WILL BE IN – NEAR 35 AND I'D LIKE TO HAVE NICE HOUSE A HOUSE THATS DONE INSIDE THAT IS A ACTIVE SOLER ELMENT IN BUILT INTO THAT AND THERE MIGHT BE A WIFE AND LADS I'D BE WORKING IN A WHITE COLLER JOB WITHIN A LABOR-LABTORY – BUPENT OR SOMETHING. MAKING 40,000 A YEAR. THE, THAT THEY – IT WOULD PUT ME INTO THE UPPER MIDDLE SOCIAL SOCIAL CLASS AND KIDS THAT I'D HAD AT THE HOME WOULD GO TO A PRIVATE SCHOOL NEAR HERE.

Figure 4.1. Chip's evaluation results and oral syntax sample.

problems in syntax are apparent across Chip's oral and written language samples. However, on measures of listening and reading comprehension, he performs above average. The problem is expressive not receptive in nature. Compare Chip's oral and written language to Betty's writing (Figure 4.3). Betty demonstrates both a receptive and expressive syntax disorder. Therefore she had difficulty understanding the structures of syntax as much as expressing them in oral or written language. Syntax problems like Betty's are much more difficult to accommodate in a learning or work environment as they affect both the understanding (listening and reading) as well as expression (speaking and writing) abilities of an individual.

When I write ~~the words I~~ my hands sometime don't write hat I'm thinking. Also

what I want the paper to convay to read and mean to what I feel does'nt I write on happen very often. I've just completed two sentences. The word "read" should have and I ment to have a "er" ending, but my pen didnt what to write many words with out there endings. The word "off" has been mispelled alot of times as "of" a less frequent mistake is reversal of letters inside or in the middle of a word. When I do ~~mispe~~ misspell a word in the middle its usually with ~~vowels~~ double vowels like ea, ie, ei, ou, etc. There are ~~alot~~ concepts that cannot be convayed by words alone, ~~One of the concepts is my that sen~~ the above sentence goes no/where forget it and these one & also ~~mispl~~ misspell these, this and who & how This becomes the or these, and these often becomes this. How become who, and who becomes how. I also like the word alot which is not a word. Now that I have explained letters and word, I will go onto the sentences parts, paragraphs and final a whole paper. Thoughts for a sentence just don't fall in place but must be organized. When I write houghts jump a head leaving a slow pen and hard to write. Where one part of a sentence should be last   forget these sentence too In writing papers, I had to reverse sentence order, move sentences, and ~~no~~ sometimes move paragraphs

Figure 4.2. Chip's writing sample.

Background Information:

Betty is a 22-year-old female who has been working with vocational rehabilitation to obtain a job. She has experienced significant problems retaining jobs due to the impact of her language-based disabilities. Results of a thorough psychological examination indicated Betty demonstrated significant deficits in executive functioning, working memory, phonology, and processing speed. Betty demonstrated significant deficits across all oral language measures at the word, sentence, and text levels. Problems were also apparent on reading comprehension measures.

Writing Sample:

What a good way in teaching writing   The ex   has to be explan clear and understand by the teach and studu

The grammar is important in teaching because you have to ~~us noun~~ know where to use and how to use it in the p   place. Out lines are s   ~~im~~ important because studest can follow it and do the signment

Figure 4.3. Background information on Betty, and her writing sample.

Written Syntax Disorders

Research from the fields of linguistics, neuropsychology, and cognitive psychology has in recent decades had a profound effect on the investigation of written syntax disorders (Gregg, 1995). Early studies in written language were concerned mainly with evaluating writers' productivity and syntactic abilities by measures such as word and sentence counts (Myklebust, 1965, 1973), t-units (Hunt, 1965, 1970), and other indices of syntactic maturity and difficulty (Harris, 1977; O'Donnell, 1976). Many of these early studies were influenced by the theory of transformational generative grammar. Transformational grammar also led to research investigating the sentence-combining skills of students (Mellon, 1969; O'Hare, 1973). Sentence combining provided a limited, patterned manipulation that allowed researchers to view a writer addressing only a few syntactic options at one time (Tomlinson, 1980). O'Donnell and Hunt (1975) attempted to assess syntax through the use of a rewrite paragraph, controlling for verbosity and topic selection. Following their research, the use of a controlled rewrite paragraph became a popular method of measuring the syntactic complexity of students' written language.

Psycholinguistic models of sentence production have also contributed significantly to a better understanding of the breakdown in written syntax development. A psycholinguistic model attempts to identify the cognitive processes involved and the order in which these processes operate during sentence production. Butterworth and Howard (1987) discussed four hypotheses explored by psycholinguists to explain the breakdown of sentence production. These hypotheses were referred to as syntactical disturbance, lexical disturbance, monitoring disturbance, and control disturbance.

The evaluator analyzing the written syntax of a student might begin by recording whether errors were due to substitution, omission, addition, or insertion of words (Myklebust, 1965). In addition, it is suggested that the evaluator determine whether a pattern can be identified across classes of words (open/closed), inflectional affixes, or word order (Butterworth & Howard, 1987).

Tasks for Evaluating Written Syntax

The assessment of written syntax should include tasks that allow the examiner to explore the student's receptive (identification) and expressive (production) syntax. Gregg and Mather (in press) developed several checklists to aid teachers in comparing oral, reading, and written language abilities of writers. The process might begin by first comparing a student's oral and written syntax competence. An examiner would need to factor out oral language differences (dialect, style) from language disorders impacting syntactic maturity. Formats that could be used in the assessment of written syntax include sentence combining, controlled stimulus passages, identification, and spontaneous writing samples. These tasks, described in the following sections, are suggested to be used in investigating a student's written syntax abilities since they require the integration of different cognitive and linguistic systems. (See Table 4.1 for a list of behaviors to observe in written text.)

Sentence Combining

Sentence combining as an evaluation measure of syntactic maturity allows the examiner to observe a student's ability to manipulate language in order to improve the maturity of syntactic structures. The student is given sets of kernel sentences, which they must combine and then write as a single complex statement. Exercises may contain grammatical cues (Mellon, 1969), nongrammatical cues (O'Hare, 1973), or no cues (Strong, 1973). In analyzing such exercises, the examiner would need to determine the types of errors (substitution, omission, addition, or insertion), classes of words, word endings, or word order that most often caused the writer difficulty.

Controlled Stimulus Passage

A controlled stimulus passage (O'Donnell & Hunt, 1975) attempts to measure the syntactic complexity of a student's writing by controlling such writing

Table 4.1
Written Syntax Disorders (Behaviors To Observe in Written Text)

Word omissions

Word order errors

Incorrect verb and pronoun use

Word ending errors

Lack of punctuation

Lack of capitalization

Discrepancy between oral and written language

Metalinguistic problems

Problems with cohesion

Problem with audience sensitivity

variables as topic, verbosity, and lack of knowledge. The student is asked to rewrite a paragraph that contains short, choppy sentences. Such a task is similar to sentence combining with the exception that the student must make decisions as to which sentences to combine or which to eliminate. Syntax, mechanical, organizational, and spelling errors should be noted by the evaluator and compared to performance across other tasks. In addition, the examiner should categorize errors by class and type.

Spontaneous Writing

Several samples of a student's spontaneous writing should be reviewed when evaluating sentence production. The evaluator will want to compare syntax competence across genre (narrative, expository), complexity of stimuli requirements (descriptive, abstract), the student's subject knowledge, and time allotted for the task. Again, an examination of types of errors and word classes most often noted as problematic for the student should be compared across performance on other tasks.

Identification

A student's understanding of syntax rules should be explored through identification as well as production tasks. Multiple-choice, word usage, punctuation, and style subtests on many achievement measures provide such tasks. This information should be compared to the individual's spontaneous writing samples. In particular, recognition and judgment of grammaticality and classification and categorization of structures should be examined. Other tasks, such as cloze passages (sentence, text), scrambled sentences, and sentence building, provide additional formats for the examiner to investigate an individual's written syntax abilities.

Relationship of Punctuation Errors to Written Syntax Disorders

Many writers with developmental writing disorders demonstrate difficulty learning and applying the rules of capitalization and punctuation. The relationship of syntactic disorders to punctuation errors has been discussed by Johnson (1987), Shaughnessy (1977), and Vogel (1986). Specific cognitive processing deficits impact a writer's ability to acquire and/or produce the rules applicable to the formulation of ideas within sentences and the assigning of appropriate punctuation. An evaluator should not ignore mechanical errors, for they are often signals of more significant morphological or syntactical deficits. At the very least, mechanical errors limit the overall semantic, syntactic, or pragmatic coherence of a piece of writing. Punctuation is integral to a writer's ability to structure meaning at the sentence and text levels. Unfortunately, process approaches to writing, such as the Hayes and Flower (1980) model, assign a very peripheral role to the understanding and application of punctuation rules.

Awareness and use of punctuation is, for the writer, a developmental process dependent to a great extent upon exposure to print. Just as invented spellings are used by children (Bissex, 1980; Read, 1975) in their beginning writing, invented punctuation is a normal stage of development (Martens & Goodman, 1996). For instance, Cordeiro (1998) found that children go through six developmental steps in learning period placement: interword, intraword, endline, endpage, endstory, and phrase structure. Invented spellings and punctuation provide opportunities for a teacher to observe students postulating rules of language (Laminack, 1991). The development of punctuation in young writers occurs as they begin to use the alphabetic principle for spelling standardization (Ferreiro & Zucchermagli, 1996). As Ferreiro and Zucchermagli (1996) noted, "Children are very sensitive to the textual functions of punctuation marks, sometimes using punctuation as an alternative means to other lexical and textual solutions" (p. 204). Many young children find punctuation marks "alien to the main principle of an alphabetic writing system" (p. 171). Learning to deal with the relationship between the graphic marks called punctuation and the graphemic marks called letters is a significant developmental step for beginning writers. Writers with underlying phonological and orthographic deficits are at high risk for difficulty grasping the complexity of punctuation.

The ability to apply punctuation rules also requires a great deal of flexibility from a writer. As C. Weaver (1998) noted, "Punctuation is, in effect, an ad hoc language process in which the rules change each time we build a new structure in writing" (p. 37). Writers who exhibit problems with inductive reasoning, therefore, will experience significant difficulties generalizing punctuation rules.

Amanda's writing sample (Figure 4.4) is an example of a young writer demonstrating significant underachievement in reading due to underlying orthographic problems. Her use of punctuation reflects her difficulty with reading. Notice how Amanda places punctuation within word and sentence boundaries.

Instructional Strategies for Written Syntax

The instruction directed at improving a student's ability to produce written syntax should begin only after thorough diagnostic assessment in order to identify specific teaching objectives. Introduction of linguistic concepts

Age: 11

Grade: 4

Psychometric Data:

Wechsler Intelligence Scale for Children–Third Edition (Wechsler, 1991)
　　Verbal Scale Score = 94
　　Performance Scale Score = 115
　　Full Scale Score = 103

Woodcock–Johnson–Revised Tests of Achievement (Woodcock & Johnson, 1989)
　　Passage Comprehension = 75 Standard Score
　　Letter Word = 56 Standard Score
　　Writing Sample = 63 Standard Score
　　Writing Fluency = 52 Standard Score
　　Listening Comprehension = 98 Standard Score
　　Calculation = 102 Standard Score
　　Applied Problems = 100 Standard Score

Writing Sample:

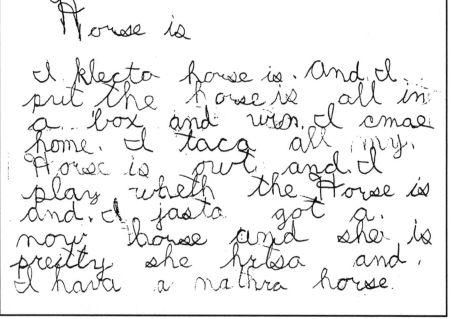

Figure 4.4. Amanda's writing sample.

should follow normal developmental guidelines outlined in such texts as Wiig and Semel (1984). Systematic practice and review related to linguistic concepts taught are integral to a writer's curriculum. Review of a writer's oral language and reading and written language goals should also be completed prior to teaching. The teacher will need to be careful that the linguistic structures introduced in a reading text are at the approximate level expected of the student in written expression tasks. The reading text(s) used by a student will greatly impact his or her style and flexibility with specific linguistic structures.

The teaching of syntax (including grammar and punctuation) rules appears to be best accomplished implicitly through the context of their use, rather than explicitly and out of context. Recent research supports the idea that "less is more" in relation to syntax and grammar rule acquisition (Noguchi, 1991; C. Weaver, 1996). Using a "scope, not sequence chart" approach, C. Weaver (1996) provided five basic grammar concepts that she considered essential to the acquisition of minimal grammar competence. Based on her research, mastery of English does not require the teaching of a complete grammatical system; rather, it depends on knowledge of five basic grammatical concepts. Her pedagogical approach addresses each of the five areas: teaching concepts such as subject, verb, sentence, phrase, and related concepts for editing; teaching style through sentence combining and sentence generating; teaching sentence style through manipulation of syntactic elements; teaching the power of dialects; and teaching punctuation, mechanics for convention, clarity, and style.

Little research can be found in the literature to support the explicit teaching of grammar rules as a means of improving composition skills. In general, the teaching of grammar in isolation does not serve any practical purpose (Hillocks, 1986; Hillocks & Smith, 1991). Yet this finding should be interpreted cautiously since the majority of research on the teaching of grammatical structures has been done with normally achieving students, not those individuals with developmental disorders. Many language arts textbooks used in the public schools introduce far too many grammatical concepts at one time or are very ambiguous about rule knowledge when teaching written language to students with developmental writing disorders. For students with written syntax problems, the introduction of grammatical concepts will require direct teaching, introduction of concepts in an organized and sequential manner, immediate feedback, modeling, and systematic practice. Yet direct teaching does not mean drill and practice on grammar rules. The writing curriculum developed for students with writing disorders might feature implicit development of grammatical awareness through such activities as sentence combining or controlled stimulus passages. Activities should range from highly structured exercises to those with less structure. (See Table 4.2 for a list of suggested instructional strategies to improve grammatical competencies.) However, grammar knowledge impacts not just at the sentence level but also at the word and text level. Instruction designed to address grammatical competence across word, sentence, and passage levels is important to writers with developmental writing disorders.

Grammar of Words

The literature related to spelling development has concentrated on the phonological and orthographic skills necessary for developing spelling. The rules related to the spelling of morphemes that tell us about the grammatical status of words has received very little attention by researchers. Nunes, Bryant, and Bindman (1997) proposed that, at specific stages, "children come to grips with the spelling of morphemes and that this new development is

Table 4.2
Written Syntax Instructional Activities

Activity	Written Syntax Instruction
High Structured Activities	Phelps Sentence Guide (Phelps-Gunn & Phelps-Terasaki, 1982)
	Controlled Stimulus Writing
	Sentence Combining (Strong, 1973)
	Sentence Expanding
	Power Writing (Sparks, 1982)
	Sentence Unscrambling (Killgallon, 1998)
	Sentence Imitating (Killgallon, 1998)
	Editing Workshops (Rosen, 1998)
	Modeling (Cramar, 1978)
	Individual Editing Conferences (Graves, 1983)
	Self-Editing Checklists (Brinkley, 1998)
Low Structured Activities	Comparison Poems (Peterson, 1998)
	Color Poems (Peterson, 1998)
	Adjective/Verb Poems (Peterson, 1998)
	Haiku
	Spontaneous Writing Across Different Genre

based on the grammatical, or, more specifically, on their morphosyntactic awareness" (p. 155). For instance, at some point of development, a young writer grasps that certain words end in –*ed* because they are past-tense verbs. It is the contention of Nunes et al. that writers undergo a shift from dependence on letter–sound correspondence to more of an awareness of grammatical structure that significantly impacts spelling success. Evidence of difficulty learning written morphological rules among writers with learning disabilities has also been observed by researchers (Carlisle, 1994, 1996; Johnson & Grant, 1989). Yet, as Carlisle (1996) noted, "Clearly, not all errors are the result of inadequate linguistic development" (p. 71). Diagnosticians and teachers sensitive to the importance of morphosyntactic ability in spelling might look for connections between a writer's syntactic skills across words, sentences, and passages, adjusting instruction accordingly.

Grammar of Passages

Competence with grammar rules entails more than just the ability to sequence words within sentences. It requires the ability to understand the grammar of passages. Mina Shaughnessy (1977) expressed this idea in *Errors and Expectations:*

> The mature writer is recognized not so much by the quality of his individual sentences as by his ability to relate sentences in such a way as to create a flow of sentences, a pattern of thought that is produced, one suspects, according to the principles of yet another kind of grammar—the grammar, let us say, of passages. (p. 226)

Cohesion and cohesive harmony are linguistic concepts that help us to better understand and address the connections between sentences and ideas in order to ascertain the grammar of passages.

Cohesion

Researchers have stated that syntagmatic approaches to studies of written language do not address the issue of the meaning of sentences. Halliday's (1978) theory suggests a fruitful way of conceptualizing the evaluation of writing. He proposed that the textual function in writing depends on cohesion both within and between sentences. Halliday and Hasan (1976) defined cohesion as the structures beyond the sentence level that establish language as a particular type of text.

Halliday and Hasan (1976) suggested that examining surface features of an individual's writing as manifestations of communication intention can lead to new insights about that student's writing. As Litowitz (1981) noted, "difficulty with cohesive devices may reflect problems with the linguistic devices themselves, the writer's sense of audience, and the actual cognitive demands of the textual structure" (p. 84).

Gregg (1985) modified the Halliday and Hasan (1976) scale of cohesion to include three basic cohesive ties: grammar ties, transitional ties, and lexical ties. Grammatical ties include any pronominal, demonstrative, or comparative terms that refer to a noun or pronoun in another sentence or paragraph. This category of ties also includes words substituted for others, or words dependent on previous sentences for their meaning. Transitional ties are words and phrases showing relationships between statements. These include what Halliday and Hasan called conjunctive ties (*and, but, therefore, however, first*). The category of lexical ties includes both reiteration and collocation ties. Reiteration ties occur when the same word is used more than once within a text; other examples include the use of synonyms and superordinate ties. Collocation ties are "achieved through the association of lexical items that regularly co-occur," such as *bread and butter* or *salt and pepper* (Halliday & Hasan, 1976, p. 284).

Researchers have found that many writers with developmental writing disorders demonstrate difficulty understanding and utilizing cohesive ties (Gregg, 1985; Wiig & Semel, 1976, 1984). Gregg (1985) found that college writers with learning disabilities used fewer demonstratives in their expository and rewrite tasks. She noted a high percentage of substitution and ellipsis ties used by these writers. Such a pattern might be due to the use of more nonspecific words than specific synonyms by writers with learning disabilities. Difficulty with word-finding could also have contributed to the overuse of general terms and common words. The absence or incorrect use of specific cohesive ties can occur for many different reasons. A close comparison of a writer's oral and written language is always imperative in determining constraints impacting performance. A diagnostician or teacher evaluating a writer's ability to utilize transitional ties might look carefully at the accuracy of transitional ties. Although a writer with developmental writing disorders might utilize a number of ties, a large percentage may be inaccurately used in the context of the meaning of the sentence or text. The student might lack the conceptual understanding behind the meaning of such tools as "time/place" and "contrast" ties (for further discussion, see Gregg, 1985). The inability to utilize lexical ties frequently and accurately can be the result of a variety of constraints.

Weaknesses with conceptual organizational strategies might be interfering with a writer's understanding of word meaning; for example, word-finding, phonological skills, and morphosyntactic awareness all contribute to accurate word retrieval, another potential constraint. Theorists have stressed that the problem of learning lies not in the storage of words, but in their retrieval, and that the key to retrieval is organization and form (Bruner, 1968; Miller, 1965). Through direct instruction of cohesion, teachers can begin to heighten a writer's awareness of both inter- and intrasentence and paragraph structures. The structure will aid meaning and the meaning will aid structure (Gregg, 1985). As Berthoff (1982) stated so well, "Form finds form" (p. 43).

Cohesive Harmony

Hasan (1984) went on to extend the earlier research she conducted with Halliday to develop the concept of cohesive harmony. While cohesion refers to the semantic bonds formed between words in a text, cohesive chaining results when there is repeated use of linguistic devices (nouns, verbs) that denote a series of actions. Therefore, cohesive harmony refers to the interaction between noun/pronoun chains and verb chains (Halliday & Hasan, 1980). "Interaction among the chains weaves the threads of meaning together into a coherent whole" (Hedberg & Fink, 1996). Cohesive harmony analysis helps in assessing a writer's ability to develop a story center focusing on a main character and a chain of events. Such an analysis can be applied to any text genre (for a complete description of cohesive harmony, see Hedberg & Westby, 1993).

Written Text Structure

The concept of text discourse and its relationship to thought and language is currently at the forefront of research in cognitive psychology. Discourse theorists have attempted to integrate linguistic, psychological, and cultural research in order to heighten understanding of the processes involved in the production of written language, and particularly in the development of form. A primary goal of the composing process is the production of coherent form (Scinto, 1982). Much of form in written language is generated through cohesion and coherence. Witte and Faigley (1981) differentiated these terms in the following manner: "Cohesion defines those underlying semantic relations that allow a text to be understood and used and coherence conditions are governed by the writer's purpose, the audiences' knowledge and expectations, and information to be conveyed" (p. 201). Therefore, investigating text organization requires an evaluation of writers' between-sentence (cohesion) relationships as well as the total form (coherence) of their writing. Coherence is the communication relationship between readers and writers, a "relationship which takes form as the intendedness of that integration or wholeness" (Phelps, 1985, p. 21).

The ability to organize ideas and arrange them to create an organizational plan involves many linguistic and cognitive skills (Scardamalia & Bereiter, 1986). Writers' cognitive development has been found to have a strong correspondence with the ability to create literary patterns (Applebee, 1978). "An awareness of text structure serves as a map that helps writers decide what information to include, and what signals (i.e., key words such as 'in contrast', 'but', 'like', 'different') to use to indicate the location of particular information" (Englert & Raphael, 1988, p. 514). The cause of a breakdown in the construction of text can be the result of many components. Therefore, an individual's ability to produce written text should be evaluated with consideration of the type of genre (narrative, expository, persuasive, descriptive); the age of the individual; the reasoning ability of the writer; the reading ability of the writer; and the writer's knowledge of the topic. A comparison is also necessary across the writer's written syntax, intraparagraph organization, and interparagraph organization.

Narrative Structure

Narratives are a genre important to success in many classroom activities (storytelling, sharing), particularly in the early elementary grades. The family of narratives encompasses scripts, recounts, accounts, events, and fictional stories (Heath, 1986; Hedberg & Westby, 1993; Hicks, 1991). The ability to understand or produce narrative requires knowledge of content, social problem solving, story, and structure (Hudson & Shapiro, 1991).

Applebee (1978) applied Vygotsky's (1962) theory of concept development to narrative-level analysis. He described six major narrative structure patterns in which children organize their stories: heaps, sequences, primitive narratives, unfocused chains, focused chains, and narratives (see Table 4.3). Applebee (1978) also found that young storytellers between the ages of 2 and 5 use the following formal conventions in their writing: a title or opening, a formal closing, and the past tense. Applebee's narrative-level analysis is very useful for the professional evaluation of the written language of students with developmental writing disorders, because many of these writers have been shown to have difficulty categorizing and organizing ideas (Englert, 1990; Englert & Raphael, 1988). However, Applebee's narrative analysis does not provide information regarding the functions of story and how one develops story plot (Hedberg & Westby, 1993). Figure 4.5 provides examples taken from children's writing and applying Applebee's narrative analysis.

Story grammars address the functions and interrelationships of ideas that create narrative structures. Stein and Glenn's (1979) story grammar, an adaptation of Labov's (1972) story analysis method, has been used quite frequently in the literature to investigate the oral and written discourse of indi-

Table 4.3

Narrative Analysis

Level	Description
Heaps	Unrelated statements Descriptions of object in the environment Declarative sentences Present or present progressive tense
Sequences	Focus on one central idea Repeated reference to one thing Organization based on shared perceptual attributes *And* only conjunction applied
Primitive narratives	Abstract relationships basis of organization Co-occurring events link to central idea Inferencing used
Unfocused chains	Temporal relationships linking to each other Causal relationships Partially structured episodes No central focus
Focused chains	Chain of events Temporal events Central idea present
Narratives	Conceptual center Strong story schema

Note. Adapted from Applebee (1978), Hedberg and Westby (1993), and Westby (1984).

viduals. Their story grammar consists of seven topologies: (1) a major setting describing the protagonist; (2) a minor setting describing the time and place of the story; (3) initiating events representing the problem that gets the story going and evokes the formation of the goals; (4) internal response indicating how the person feels about the initiating event (internal responses also serve as the motivation for later action); (5) actions that are attempts at meeting the goals; (6) direct consequences indicating whether or not the goal was attained; and (7) reactions that include a character's feelings or thoughts about the outcome and how characters are affected by the outcome. Such a topology, while only appropriate, for narrative types of discourse, has been used frequently by teachers and researchers evaluating the written language of students with developmental writing disorders. One does need, however, to be very careful in using story grammars when analyzing the writing of learners with developmental writing disorders. As Hedberg and

---

Sample 1: Grade: 2
        Age: 8
        Heaps Level

I like To be Lois Lane
I like To be a Dog
I like to be a indian
I like to be the Welcome
I like to be Miss BS

Sample 2: Grade: 2
        Age: 7
        Sequence Level

If I were a pumpkin
I wod go and look arood
And go to see my fresars
Then go to Mrs. Rees and to see
Mre Burguss.

Sample 3: Grade: 2
        Age: 8
        Primitive Narrative

Wen I was little I did no no
better and I wos messing
hith a dog then he
chased me and I ran to
my master's/I looked out
the window and saw
some body and I started
scratching the door to give my
master's a warning that some
body is at the door/I hope
I am a good cat/good
bay

Sample 4: Grade: 3
        Age: 8
        Unfocused

My life in day of a cat
I would lay in the window
and rest. then I would wake
up and eat my cat foot
then I would lay on my
master's lap and let him
rub my back./Then I
would make sure there are
no rats or mice in the house
Then I would go outside
and play with my yarn and
get my friend/some time I
Will ride in the car with my
master's we go to get some cat food

Figure 4.5. Applebee's (1978) narrative analysis applied to writing samples.

Westby (1993) stated, "Persons with language disorders, however, frequently begin a story with an appropriate setting and initiating event that triggers a goal, but then they begin to chain actions and reactions together with little or no thought of the goal that had been implicitly or even explicitly stated" (p. 135). Story grammars can have limited diagnostic utility due to their relative insensitivity to developmental disorders (P. A. Weaver & Dickinson, 1982). The usefulness of story grammars is dependent upon the skill of the diagnostician.

Expository

The expository genre involves reflections of experiences common to many people or an entire culture rather than the reflection of a single person (narrative). As Hedberg and Westby (1993) noted, "Expository school texts represent the ultimate in distancing and generalizing" (p. 10). Expository discourse becomes more integrated into the school curriculum as children progress through the grades. The family of expository texts includes explanations (sequences), comparisons/contrasts, descriptions, and enumerations or expert text forms (Englert, 1990; Meyer, 1975; Meyer, Brandt, & Bluth, 1980). Many students with written developmental disorders have difficulty with the text structures in expository text (Englert, Raphael, Anderson, Gregg, & Anthony, 1989; Englert & Thomas, 1987). Difficulties have been noted with the ability of such students to employ self-directed memory searches to retrieve text schemes (Englert & Raphael, 1988).

The importance of self-regulation to the writing process has been the focus of much recent research exploring the production of expository text (Berninger, 1999; Graham, 1997, 1999). Englert (1990) observed that self-talk or self-regulation impacts planning, organizing, drafting, and editing. Many writers with developmental writing disorders appear inadequately aware of writing strategies, and more important, are insufficiently sensitive at times to their audience (Englert, 1990; Englert & Raphael, 1989; Englert et al., 1989; Gregg & McAlexander, 1989; Gregg, Sigalas, Hoy, Wisenbaker, & McKinley, 1996).

Buzz is an example of an adolescent writer with learning disabilities and attention-deficit/hyperactivity disorder. The impact of speed of processing, attention, executive functioning (self-regulation and planning), and working memory deficits impact his ability to organize, revise, and maintain a sense of audience when asked to write about his worst day (see Figures 4.6 and 4.7).

Sense of Audience

A sense of audience requires the writer to make the necessary adjustments and choices necessary to meet the needs of the intended reader(s). A writer's ability to identify and remain sensitive to a specific audience influences almost every aspect of written composition. Students who demonstrate little audience awareness often supply few details or elaboration of their ideas (Flower, 1979; Shaughnessy, 1977). The manner in which writers organize their texts has also been found to be dependent on audience awareness (Berkenkotter, 1981; Flower, 1979). Several researchers have discovered that the choice of syntactic structures is audience dependent (Crowhurst & Piche, 1979; Rubin, 1982; Smith & Swan, 1978). Shaughnessy (1977) pointed out

Age: 15 years old
Grade: 9th grade

Background:

Buzz was diagnosed with learning disabilities and attention-deficit/hyperactivity disorder in first grade. He received support through both self-contained and pull-out programs (resource) throughout his schooling. Transitional plans are currently being written for Buzz.

Psychometric Data:

Wechsler Intelligence Scale for Children–Third Edition (Wechsler, 1991)

Verbal Scale Score = 86
Performance Scale Score = 81
Full Scale Score = 82

Woodcock–Johnson–Revised Tests of Achievement (Woodcock & Johnson, 1989)

CLUSTER/Test	SS	SS 68% BAND
BCA (Std)	78	75–81
S-T MEM (Gsm)	86	81–91
PROC SPEED (Gs)	65	59–71
AUD PROC (Ga)	129	124–134
COMP-KNOW (Gc)	88	84–92
FLUID REAS (Gf)	88	85–91
READING APT	88	85–91
MATHEMATICS APT	78	75–81
BROAD READING	100	96–104
READING SKILLS	113	110–116
BROAD MATH (Gq)	77	74–80
MATH REASONING	80	76–84
Memory Names	69	65–73
Memory Sents	90	84–96
Visual Matching	69	63–75
Inc Words	112	105–119
Visual Closure	93	86–100
Picture Vocab	91	86–96
Analysis-Synth	82	79–86
Memory Words	86	79–93
Cross Out	73	66–80
Sound Blending	132	126–138
Oral Vocab	88	83–93
Concept Form	89	85–93
Numbers Rev	67	63–71
Spatial Rels	91	85–97
Verbal Angls	84	80–88
L-W Ident	118	114–122
Passage Comp	89	84–94
Calculation	76	72–80
Applied Probs	80	76–84
Word Attack	103	98–108

Figure 4.6. Buzz's background and evaluation results.

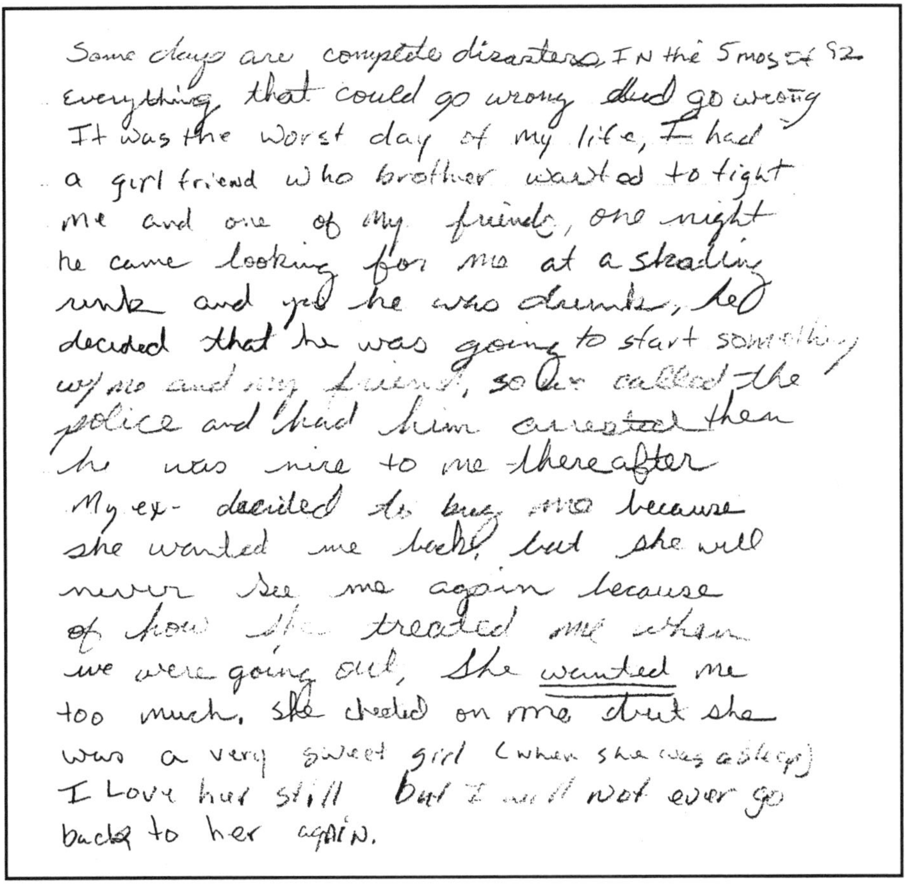

Some days are complete disasters IN the 5 mos of 92.
everything that could go wrong did go wrong
It was the worst day of my life, I had
a girl friend who brother wanted to fight
me and one of my friends, one night
he came looking for me at a skating
rink and yet he who drunks, he
decided that he was going to start something
w/ me and my friend, so I called the
police and had him arrested then
he was nice to me thereafter.
My ex- decided to buy me because
she wanted me back, but she will
never see me again because
of how she treated me when
we were going out, she wanted me
too much, she cheated on me but she
was a very sweet girl (when she was asleep)
I Love her still but I will not ever go
back to her again.

Figure 4.7. Buzz's writing sample.

several years ago that ambiguous pronoun reference is often the result of a writer's inability to take the reader's perspective.

Assessment and Instructional Strategies for Written Text Structure

Concern for developing a measure that would evaluate writing from the point of view of the total discourse led to the development of the holistic score. The Educational Testing Service first coined the term *holistic* to define a type of scoring of written language that can be done in a quick and reliable manner (Vogel & Moran, 1982). It is an impressionistic evaluation of writing that looks at the total text and sorts and ranks ratings in a guided procedure. The principle underlying holistic scoring is that writing is communication; that is, the intended message of the writer (i.e., meaning) must not be fragmented such that the whole is diminished. Yet holistic scoring does not provide the evaluator with any detailed information or error analysis about a writer's abilities (Spandel & Stiginnis, 1990).

Analytic or primary-trait scoring is a form of holistic scoring that produces a more detailed analysis of writing while keeping the same holistic evaluation philosophy. A scale is developed to assign points to the different levels of performance that a person is interested in evaluating (Gregg et al., 1996).

Englert's (1990) Cognitive Strategy in Writing (CSIW) curriculum also provides teachers with an opportunity to integrate evaluation and instruction together in an authentic manner. The strategies underlying CSIW that indicate the ability to plan, organize, write, edit, and revise are key to producing text. These strategies were identified from the literature as those that skilled writers employ (Bruce, Collin, Rubin, & Gentner, 1982; Hayes & Flower, 1980). Evaluation of strategy use should be conducted in the context of the writing assignment. Therefore, in order to assess a student's explanation paper, an analytic or primary-trait scale could be designed that would indicate the student's use of an introduction, steps in the explanation, use of key words, and overall organization. For an assignment requiring the writer to produce what Englert et al. (1989) called the expert paper, an analytic scale would need to include items for introduction, definition of categories, development within categories (depth), development across categories, keywords, and organization (Hallenbeck, 1996). In addition, both audience sensitivity and text organization should always be examined. Observations of how the writer preplans, edits, and revises during the writing process are also invaluable to an instructor.

The results of an evaluation of a writer's ability to plan, organize, write, edit, and revise would lead to an individualized instructional plan. The curriculum material created by Englert (1990) for the CSIW included think-sheets designed to heighten a writer's awareness of writing strategies, self-talk, and text structures (for a complete description of CSIW curriculum, see Englert, 1990; Raphael & Englert, 1990). Visual think-sheets free writers from trying to remember the self-questions and strategies for generating text. The CSIW curriculum includes think-sheets for planning, organizing, self-editing, and editing for others. While the visual think-sheets are essential to the CSIW curriculum, they must not be seen as the only key to the success of this program. The emphasis of the CSIW is on providing dialogue, modeling, scaffolding, and generalization activities. These same instructional components are critical to the teaching of syntax as well as text structure. Englert (1990) aptly summarized the success of the CSIW: "It is the teacher's insightful modeling and demonstration that activates students to become more proficient informants and strategic problem solvers into the expository writing process" (p. 221). While Englert's research has focused on elementary-age children, Hallenbeck (1996) successfully modified the CSIW for use with the adolescent population and incorporated the use of computers.

Other effective instructional methods for enhancing written text expression include free writing (Elbow, 1973), story frames (Cudd & Roberts, 1987), semantic mapping (Sinatra, Stahl-Gemake, & Morgan, 1986), dialogue journals, and metalinguistic checklists. Software programs such as *Writer's Helper* (1997) and *Inspiration* (Helfgott, Helfgott, & Hoof, 1993) provide excellent activities addressing the development of sentence and text organization.

Future Directions

Vygotksy (1962) discussed the complex process of writing and postulated that learning to write involves mastery of cognitive skills within the development of new social understanding. He felt we categorize and synthesize our lives through inner speech—the language of thought. Transforming one's inner language into written text requires one to step outside of his or her own perspective in order to enter the social context of the reader. Therefore, writing involves not only knowledge of the topic, rhetorical knowledge, and metacommunication skills (Burleson, 1984), but also an awareness of the intended audience (reader) and a sensitivity to the reader's needs. Indeed, coherence and cohesion in writing result in a large part from intentions that are appropriate to a specified audience. Thus, audience awareness must be coupled with genre competence to allow a writer to be effective in communicating ideas. More research is certainly needed to determine the impact of various developmental disabilities on the writing process. Forthcoming will be an example of how written expression was impacted by two writers' learning and behavior disorders.

 Tim

Tim is a 15-year-old freshman at a rural high school and is classified as demonstrating specific learning disabilities and behavior disorders. Tim has recently been in trouble with the local authorities for shoplifting. On average, he misses school 2 days per week due to placement in either in-school suspension or suspension at home. Teachers report many inappropriate school behaviors, such as talking out, tardiness, lack of effort, refusing to work, failure to turn in assignments, and rudeness to teachers.

Tim achieved average scores on measures of the *Wechsler Intelligence Scale for Children–Third Edition* (Wechsler, 1991), with his Performance Scale score falling 9 points higher than his Verbal Scale score. He speaks with a Black English dialect and refers to himself as being "streetwise." On the *Oral and Written Language Scales* (Carrow-Woolfolk, 1995), he obtained low average on the Listening Comprehension Scale and below average on the Oral Expression Scale. Reading scores were predominately below average. On the *Woodcock–Johnson–Revised Tests of Achievement* (WJ–R) (Woodcock & Johnson, 1989), Tim obtained standard scores of 62 on the Word Attack subtest (nonsense words), 85 on the Letter–Word subtest (real words), and 79 on Passage Comprehension. Additional phonological and orthographic skills were assessed using informal tools. Tim's orthographic abilities appeared to be stronger than his phonological, with phonological segmentation skills being the most significant area of underachievement. Written language standard scores were all below average. Tim obtained a 73 standard score on the WJ–R Writing Sample subtest and a 61 on the Writing Fluency subtest.

Tim's writing sample (see Figure 4.8) provides clear examples of spelling, punctuation, capitalization, subject/verb agreement, format, use of contractions, omission of word endings, insufficient development of ideas, and sense of audience. Tim was attempting to write a letter of application for a job to a rap group. He used an incorrect format for a business letter and used infor-

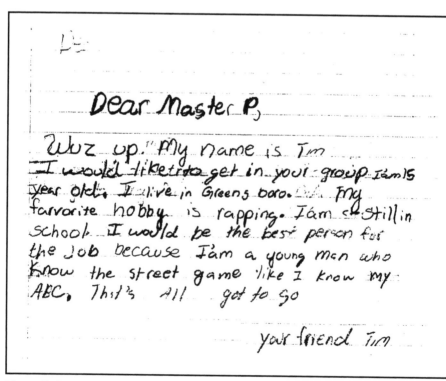

Figure 4.8. Tim's writing sample.

mal "street" jargon. His social identity is strongly associated with the language of his age group and cultural community. His sentences were short and choppy, and the information about himself he provided in the letter was inadequate for a letter of application. Organization of his ideas and taking the perspective of his audience were also problematic.

Billy

Billy attends the same rural high school as Tim, is in the ninth grade, and demonstrates a specific learning disability. He does not have a history of behavior problems, although he has always struggled academically in school. Billy is involved with the track team and practices daily after school. His writing sample concerns this interest and his involvement (see Figure 4.9).

Billy's scores on the WISC–III (Wechsler, 1991) in the low average range with performance at a 95 and verbal at a 79 scaled score. On the *Oral and Written Language Scales* (Carrow-Woolfolk, 1995), he obtained a 62 scaled score on the Listening Comprehension Scale and a 75 scaled score on the Oral Expression scale. On the WJ–R Word Attack subtest (nonsense words), Billy obtained a standard score of 59. On the Letter–Word and Passage Comprehension subtests of the WJ–R, he received standard scores of 75 and 62, respectively. Additional phonological and orthographic skills were assessed using informal tools. Billy's phonological and orthographic skills were both significantly below average for his age and ability. Written language standard scores were all below average. Tim obtained a 65 standard score on the WJ–R Writing Sample subtest and a 61 on the Writing Fluency subtest.

The writing sample for Billy contains numerous errors in spelling, punctuation, and capitalization. His writing is replete with run-on sentences and sentence fragments. His ideas are jumbled and insufficiently developed. Problems with word usage, subject–verb agreement, and organization are also apparent. In the second half of the sample, Billy attempted to write about his religious beliefs and his prayers, but information is omitted and meaning is disturbed. His social identity is strongly associated with his religion. He appears to have limited awareness of the need of his audience, but instead assumes readers will have information concerning the track team, the track coach, and Billy's successes and failures in track.

Case Studies: Summary

The writing samples discussed are typical of many students with developmental written expression disorders. Neither student appears to have used preplanning, revising, or editing strategies in composing the text. Both pupils exhibited low achievement scores in reading and written expression. They also demonstrated similar problems with mechanics, organization (sentence and text), and audience awareness. Billy and Tim display significant deficits in the area of written communication.

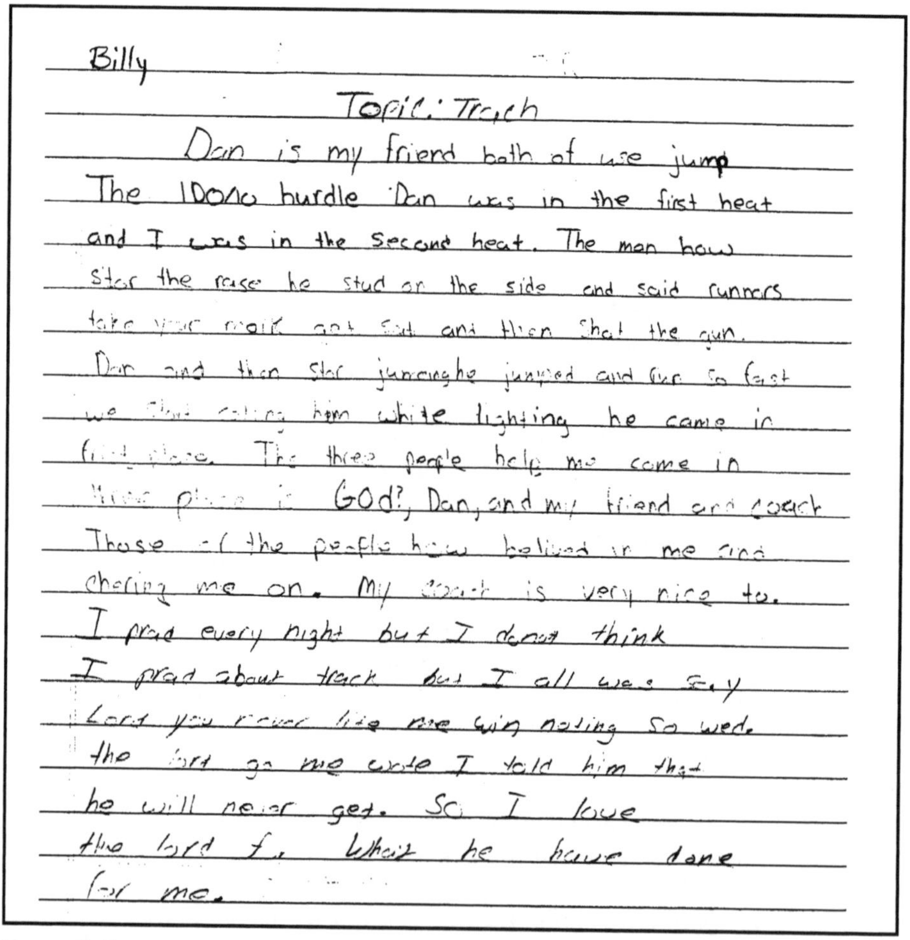

Figure 4.9. Billy's writing sample.

References

Applebee, A. N. (1978). *The child's concept of a story*. Chicago: University of Chicago Press.

Berkenkotter, C. (1981). Understanding a writer's awareness of audience. *College Composition and Communication, 32,* 388–399.

Berninger, V. W. (1996). *Reading and writing acquisition: A developmental neuropsychological perspective*. New York: Westview Press.

Berninger, V. W. (1999). Coordinating transcription and text generation in working memory during composing: Automatic and constructive process. *Learning Disabilities Quarterly, 22,* 99–112.

Berninger, V., Yates, C., Cartwright, A., Rutberg, J., Remy, E., & Abbott, R. (1992). Lower-level developmental skills in beginning writing. *Reading and Writing: An Interdisciplinary Journal, 4,* 257–280.

Berthoff, A. E. (1982). *Forming, thinking, writing the composing process*. New York: Boyton Cook.

Bissex, G. (1980). *GNYS AT WRK: A child learns to write and read*. Cambridge, MA: Harvard University Press.

Blanck, G. (1990). Vygotsky: The man and his cause. In L. C. Moll (Ed.), *Vygotsky and education: Instructional implications and applications of sociohistorical psychology* (pp. 31–58). New York: Cambridge University Press.

Brinkley, E. (1998). Learning to use grammar with precision through editing conference. In C. Weaver (Ed.), *Lessons to share: On teaching grammar in context* (pp. 120–136). Portsmouth, NH: Heinemann.

Brown, A. L., & Palincsar, A. S. (1988). Reciprocal teaching of comprehensive strategies: A natural history of one program for enhancing learning. In J. Borkowski & J. P. Das (Eds.), *Intelligence and cognition in special children: Comparative shades of giftedness, mental retardation, and learning disabilities* (pp. 92–129). New York: Abler.

Bruce, B., Collin, A., Rubin, A. D., & Gentner, D. (1982). Three perspectives on writing. *Educational Psychologist, 17,* 131–145.

Bruner, J. (1968). *Towards a theory of instruction* (2nd ed.). New York: Norton.

Burleson, B. R. (1984). The affective perspective taking process: A test of Turiel's role-taking model. In M. Burleson (Ed.), *Communication yearbook II* (pp. 473–488). Beverly Hills, CA: Sage.

Butterworth, B., & Howard, D. (1987). Paragrammatisms. *Cognition, 26,* 1–37.

Carlisle, J. F. (1994). Morphological awareness, spelling and story writing: Possible relationships for elementary-age learning disabled and non learning disabled children. In N. Jordan & J. Goldsmith-Philips (Eds.), *Learning disabilities: New directions for assessment and intervention* (pp. 123–145). Needham Heights, MA: Allyn & Bacon.

Carlisle, J. F. (1996). An exploratory study of morphological errors in children's written stories. *Reading and Writing: An Interdisciplinary Journal, 8,* 61–72.

Carrow-Woolfolk, E. C. (1995). *Oral and Written Language Scales*. Circle Pines, MN: American Guidance Service.

Cordeiro, P. (1998). Dora learns to write and in the process encounters punctuation. In C. Weaver (Ed.), *Lessons to share: On teaching grammar in context* (pp. 39–66). Portsmouth, NH: Heinemann.

Cramar, R. (1978). *Children's writing and language growth*. Columbus, OH: Merrill.

Cromer, R. F. (1980). Spontaneous spelling by language-disordered children. In U. Frith (Ed.), *Cognitive processes in spelling* (pp. 402–422). London: Academic Press.

Crowhurst, M., & Piche, G. L. (1979). Audience and mode of discourse effects on syntactic complexity at two grade levels. *Research in the Teaching of English, 13,* 101–109.

Cudd, E. T., & Roberts, L. L. (1987). Using story frames to develop reading comprehension in a 1st grade classroom. *The Reading Teacher, 8,* 74–79.

Deuel, R. K., & Collins, R. C. (1984). The functional anatomy of frontal lobe neglect in the monkey: Behavioral and quantitative 2-deoxglucose studies. *Annals of Neurology, 15,* 521–529.

Elbow, P. (1973). *Writing without teachers.* New York: Oxford University Press.

Englert, C. S. (1990). Unraveling the mysteries of writing through strategy instruction. In T. E. Scruggs & B. Y. L. Wong (Eds.), *Intervention research in learning disabilities* (pp. 186–223). New York: Springer-Verlag.

Englert, C. S. (1992). Writing instruction from a sociocultural perspective: The holistic, dialogic, and social enterprise of writing. *Journal of Learning Disabilities, 6,* 153–172.

Englert, C. S., & Palincsar, A. S. (1991). Reconsidering instructional research in literacy from a sociocultural perspective. *Learning Disabilities Research and Practice, 6,* 225–229.

Englert, C. S., & Raphael, T. E. (1988). Constructing well-formed prose: Process, structure, and metacognitive knowledge. *Exceptional Children, 54,* 513–520.

Englert, C. S., & Raphael, T. E. (1989). Developing successful writers through cognitive strategy instruction. In J. E. Brophy (Ed.), *Advances in research on teaching* (Vol. 2, pp. 105–151). Greenwich, CT: JAI.

Englert, C. S., Raphael, T. E., Anderson, L. M., Gregg, S. L., & Anthony, H. M. (1989). Exposition: Reading, writing and the metacognitive knowledge of learning disabled students. *Learning Disabilities Research, 5,* 5–24.

Englert, C. S., & Thomas, C. C. (1987). Sensitivity to text structure in reading and writing: A comparison between learning disabled and non-learning disabled students. *Learning Disabilities Quarterly, 10,* 93–105.

Ferreiro, E., & Zucchermagli, C. (1996). Children's use of punctuation marks: A case of quoted speech. In C. Pontecorvo, M. Orsolini, B. Burge, & L. Resnick (Eds.), *Children's early text construction.* Mahwah, NJ: Erlbaum.

Flower, L. S. (1979). Writer-based prose: A cognitive basis for problems in writing. *College English, 41,* 19–37.

Getting, P. (1989). Emerging principles governing the operations of neural networks. *Annual Review of Neuroscience, 12,* 185–204.

Graham, S. (1997). Executive control in the revising of students with learning and writing difficulties. *Journal of Educational Psychology, 89,* 223–234.

Graham, S. (1999). The role of text production skills in writing development: A special issue. *Learning Disabilities Quarterly, 22,* 75–77.

Graham, S., Harris, K. R., MacArthur, C. A., & Schwartz, S. (1991). Writing and writing instruction for students with learning disabilities: Review of a research program. *Learning Disabilities Quarterly, 14,* 89–114.

Graham, S., & Weintraub, N. (1996). A review of handwriting research: Progress and prospects from 1980 to 1994. *Educational Psychology Review, 8,* 7–87.

Graves, D. (1983). *Writing: Teachers and children at work.* Portsmouth, NH: Heinemann.

Gregg, N. (1985). College learning disabled, normal, and basic writers: A comparison of frequency and accuracy of cohesive ties. *Journal of Psychoeducational Assessment, 3,* 223–231.

Gregg, N. (1989). Expressive writing disorders. In S. Hooper & G. Hynd (Eds.), *Assessment and diagnosis of child and adolescent psychiatric disorder: Current issues and procedures.* Hillsdale, NJ: Erlbaum.

Gregg, N. (1995). *Written expression disorders.* The Netherlands: Kluwer Academic.

Gregg, N., & Mather, N. (in press). Best thing about school is recess: Informal assessment of written language for students with learning disabilities. *Journal of Learning Disabilities.*

Gregg, N., & McAlexander, P. A. (1989). The relation between sense of audience and specific learning disabilities: An exploration. *Annals of Dyslexia, 39,* 206–226.

Gregg, N., Sigalas, S. A., Hoy, C., Wisenbaker, J., & McKinley, C. (1996). Sense of audience and the adult writer: A study across competence levels. *Reading and Writing: An Interdisciplinary Journal, 8,* 121–137.

Hallenbeck, M. J. (1996). The cognitive strategy in writing: Welcome relief for adolescents with learning disabilities. *Learning Disabilities Research and Practice, 11,* 107–119.

Halliday, M. A. K. (1978). *Language as social semiotics: The social interpretation of language and meaning.* London: University Park Press.

Halliday, M. A. K., & Hasan, R. (1976). *Cohesion in English.* London: Longman.

Halliday, M. A. K., & Hasan, R. (1980). *Text and context: Aspects of language in a social-semiotic perspective.* Tokyo: Sophia University.

Harris, M. M. (1977). Oral and written syntax attainment of second graders. *Research in the Testing of English, 11,* 117–132.

Hasan, R. (1984). Coherence and cohesive harmony. In J. Flood (Ed.), *Understanding reading comprehension* (pp. 139–154). Newark, DE: International Reading Association.

Hayes, J., & Flower, L. (1980). Identifying the organization of the writing process. In L. W. Gregg & E. R. Sternberg (Eds.), *Cognitive processes in writing* (pp. 3–30). Hillsdale, NJ: Erlbaum.

Heath, S. B. (1986). Taking a cross-cultural look at narratives. *Topics in Language Disorders, 7,* 84–94.

Hedberg, N. L., & Fink, R. J. (1996). Cohesive harmony in the written stories of elementary children. *Reading and Writing: An Interdisciplinary Journal, 8,* 73–86.

Hedberg, N. L., & Westby, C. E. (1993). *Analyzing storytelling skills: Theory to practice.* Tucson, AZ: Communication Skill Builders.

Helfgott, D., Helfgott, M., & Hoof, B. (1993). *Inspiration.* Portland, OR: Inspiration Software.

Hicks, D. (1991). Kinds of narrative: Genre skills among first graders from two communities. In A. McCabe & C. Peterson (Eds.), *Developing narrative structure* (pp. 55–87). Hillsdale, NJ: Erlbaum.

Hillocks, G. (1986). *Research on written composition: New directions for teaching.* Urbana, IL: ERIC Clearinghouse on Reading and Composition Skills and the National Conference on Research in English. Distributed by the National Council of Teachers of English.

Hillocks, G., & Smith, M. W. (1991). Grammar and usage. In J. Flood, J.M. Jensen, D. Lapp, & J. R. Squire (Eds.), *Handbook of research on teaching the English language arts* (pp. 591–603). New York: Macmillan.

Hudson, J. A., & Shapiro, L. R. (1991). From knowing to telling: The development of children's scripts, stories, and personal narratives. In A. McCabe & C. Peterson (Eds.), *Developing narrative structure* (pp. 89–136). Hillsdale, NJ: Erlbaum.

Hunt, K. W. (1965). *Grammatical structures written at three grade levels* (Research Rep. No. 3). Urbana, IL: National Council of Teachers of English.

Hunt, K. W. (1970). Syntactic maturity in children and adults. *Monographs of the Society for Research in Child Development, 35,* 25–37. Chicago: University of Chicago Press.

Johnson, D. (1987). Disorders of written language. In D. J. Johnson & J. W. Blalock (Eds.), *Adults with learning disabilities: Clinical studies* (pp. 173–203). Orlando, FL: Grune & Stratton.

Johnson, D. J., & Grant, J. O. (1989). Written narratives of normal and learning disabled students. *Annals of Dyslexia, 39,* 140–158.

Killgallon, D. (1998). Sentence composing. In C. Weaver (Ed.), *Lessons to share: On teaching grammar in context* (pp. 169–185). Portsmouth, NH: Heinemann.

Labov, W. (1972). *Language in the inner city: Studies in the black vernacular.* Philadelphia: University of Pennsylvania Press.

Laminack, L. (1991). *Learning with Zachary.* Richmond Hill, Ontario: Scholastic.

Litowitz, B. (1981). Developmental issues in written language. *Topics in Language Disorders, 1*(2), 73–89.

Luria, A. R. (1980). *Higher cortical functions in man.* New York: Basic Books.

Luria, A. R. (1981). *Language and cognition.* New York: Wiley Intersciences.

Martens, F., & Goodman, Y. (1996). Invented punctuation. In N. Hall & A. Robinson (Eds.), *Learning about punctuation.* Portsmouth, NH: Heinemann.

McCutchen, D. (1996). A capacity theory of writing: Working memory in composition. *Educational Psychology Review, 8,* 299–325.

Mellon, J. C. (1969). *Transformational sentence combining: A method for enhancing the development of syntactic fluency in English composition* (Research Rep. No. 10). Urbana, IL: National Council of Teachers of English.

Meyer, B. J. F. (1975). *The organization of prose and its effects on memory.* Amsterdam: North-Holland.

Meyer, B. J. F., Brandt, D. H., & Bluth, G. J. (1980). Use of author's textual schema: Key for ninth-graders' comprehension. *Reading Research Quarterly, 16,* 72–103.

Michaels, S., & O'Connor, M. C. (1990). *Literacy as reasoning within multiple discourses: Implications for policy and educational reform.* Paper presented at the Summer Institute of the Council of Chief State School Officers, Clark University, Newton, MA.

Miller, G. A. (1965). Computers, communication, and cognition. *Advancement of Science, 21,* 417–430.

Myklebust, H. (1965). *Development and disorders of written language* (Vol. 1). New York: Grune & Stratton.

Myklebust, H. (1973). *Development and disorders of written language: Studies of normal and exceptional children* (Vols. 1–2). New York: Grune & Stratton.

Noguchi, R. R. (1991). *Grammar and the teaching of writing: Limits and possibilities.* Urbana, IL: National Council of Teachers of English.

Nunes, T., Bryant, P., & Bindman, M. (1997). Spelling and grammar—The NECSED move. In C. A. Perfetti, L. Rieben, & M. Fayol (Eds.), *Learning to spell: Research, theory and practice across languages* (pp. 151–194). New York: Erlbaum.

O'Donnell, R. C. (1976). A critique of some indices of syntactic maturity. *Research in the Teaching of English, 10,* 31–38.

O'Donnell, R. C., & Hunt, K. (1975). Syntactic Maturity Test. In W. T. Fagan, C. R. Cooper, & J. M. Jensen (Eds.), *Measures for research and evaluation in the English language arts* (pp. 22–37). Urbana, IL: National Council of Teachers of English.

O'Hare, F. (1973). *Sentence combining: Improving student writing without formal grammar instruction* (Research Rep. No. 15). Urbana, IL: National Council of Teachers of English.

Peterson, S. (1998). Teaching writing and grammar in context. In C. Weaver (Ed.), *Lessons to share: On teaching grammar in context* (pp. 67–94). Portsmouth, NH: Heinemann.

Phelps, L. W. (1985). Dialects of coherence: Toward an integrative theory. *College English, 47*(1), 12–29.

Phelps-Gunn, T., & Phelps-Terasaki, D. (1982). *Written language instruction.* Rockville, MD: Aspen.

Raphael, T. E., & Englert, C. S. (1990). Reading and writing: Partners in constructing meaning. *The Reading Teacher, 43,* 388–400.

Read, C. (1975). *Children's categorization of speech sounds in English* (Research Rep. No. 17). Urbana, IL: National Council of Teachers of English.

Roeltgen, D. (1985). Agraphia. In K. M. Heilman & E. Valenstein (Eds.), *Clinical neuropsychology* (pp. 75–110). New York: Oxford University Press.

Rosen, L. (1998). Developing correctness in student writing: Alternatives to the error hunt. *English Journal, 76,* 62–69.

Rubin, D. L. (1982). Adapting syntax in writing to varying audiences as a function of age and social cognitive ability. *Journal of Child Language, 9,* 497–510.

Scardamalia, M., & Bereiter, C. (1986). Research on written composition. In M. C. Wittock (Ed.), *Handbook of research on teaching* (pp. 778–803). New York: Macmillan.

Scinto, L. F. M. (1982). *The acquisition of functional composition strategies for text.* Hamburg, Germany: Helmut Bushe.

Shaughnessy, M. P. (1977). *Errors and expectations: A guide for the teacher of basic writing.* New York: Oxford University Press.

Sinatra, R., Stahl-Gemake, J., & Morgan, N. W. (1986). Using semantic mapping after reading to organize and write original discourse. *Journal of Reading, 8,* 4–13.

Smith, N. L., & Swan, M. B. (1978). Adjusting syntactic structures to varied levels of audience. *Journal of Experimental Education, 46,* 29–34.

Spandel, V., & Stiginnis, R. J. (1990). *Creating writing.* New York: Longman.

Sparks, J. (1982). *Power writing.* Los Angeles: Communication Associates.

Stein, N. L., & Glenn, C. G. (1979). An analysis of story comprehension in elementary school children. In R. O. Fredle (Ed.), *Advances in discourse processing: Vol. 2. New directions in discourse processing* (pp. 27–96). Norwood, NJ: Ablex.

Strong, W. (1973). *Sentence combining: A composing book.* New York: Random House.

Tomlinson, B. M. (1980) *The influence of sentence combining instruction on the syntactic maturity and writing quality of minority college freshmen in a summer preentry preparation program.* Unpublished doctoral dissertation, University of California, Riverside.

Vogel, S. A. (1986). Syntactic complexity in written expression of LD college writers. *Annals of Dyslexia, 35,* 135–157.

Vogel, S. A., & Moran, M. (1982). Written language disorders in learning disabled college students: A preliminary report. In W. Cruickshank & J. Lerner (Eds.), *Coming of age: The best of ACLD* (Vol. 3, pp. 32–49). Syracuse, NY: Syracuse University Press.

Vygotsky, L. S. (1962). *Thought and language.* Cambridge, MA: MIT Press.

Vygotsky, L. S. (1978). *Mind and society: The development of higher psychological processes.* Cambridge, MA: Harvard University Press.

Weaver, C. (1996). *Teaching grammar in context.* Portsmouth, NH: Heinemann.

Weaver, C. (1998). Teaching grammar in the context of writing. In C. Weaver (Ed.), *Lessons to share: On teaching grammar in context* (pp. 18–38). Portsmouth, NH: Heinemann.

Weaver, P. A., & Dickinson, D. K. (1982). Scratching below the surface structure: Exploring the usefulness of story grammars. *Discourse Processes, 5,* 225–243.

Wechsler, D. (1991). *Wechsler Intelligence Scale for Children–Third Edition.* San Antonio: Psychological Corporation.

Wertsch, J.V. (1998). *Mind as action.* New York: Oxford University Press.

Westby, C. (1984). Development of narrative language abilities. In G. Wallach & K. Butler (Eds.), *Language learning disabilities in school-aged children* (pp. 103–270). Baltimore: Williams & Wilkins.

Wiig, E. H., & Semel, E. M. (1976). *Language disabilities in children and adolescents.* Columbus, OH: Merrill.

Wiig, E. H., & Semel, E. (1984). *Language assessment and intervention for the learning disabled* (2nd ed.). Columbus, OH: Merrill.

Witte, S. P., & Faigley, L. (1981). Coherence, cohesion, and writing ability. *College Composition and Communication, 32,* 189–204.

Woodcock, R. W., & Johnson, M. B. (1989). *Woodcock–Johnson–Revised Tests of Achievement.* Allen, TX: Riverside.

Writer's Helper. (Version 4.0) [Computer software]. (1997). Upper Saddle River, NJ: Prentice Hall.

More Than Words: Learning To Write in the Digital World 5

Anne Meyer, Elizabeth Murray, and Bart Pisha

Learning to write effectively is central to becoming literate. Yet learning to write is a long and complex process. Writing requires understanding and using the patterns of language; practicing and perfecting planning and expressive skills; and building confidence and motivation to persist. Students with language-processing disorders face extraordinary challenges in learning to write, but technology can be a powerful ally.

In an earlier edition of this chapter, we advocated integrating a process approach to writing instruction with selected elements of a product approach. To maximize learning, we proposed that teachers provide meaningful communication contexts for writing and individually target instruction in specific skill deficits. Within this framework, we offered examples of computer software and hardware that could support learning for students with written language disabilities.

We have revised our approach to using technology in writing instruction for students with learning disabilities because of two important developments. First, the Center for Applied Special Technology (CAST) has created a new framework called Universal Design for Learning (UDL), based on evidence from neurological research about the nature of learning. Using this framework, we focus on three critical components in teaching writing: content, strategies, and motivation. Second, the universe of personal computing as it pertains to writing has been radically remapped by technological innovation. The selection and quality of available computer systems and digital materials and tools has improved dramatically in recent years, facilitating the individualization of teaching to meet the needs of diverse learners.

We propose a model of balanced writing instruction based on new approaches to learning, teaching, and the uses of technology to support individual learning differences. Using insights from CAST's framework, we draw implications about how to apply new technologies to the teaching of writing.

We address the three aspects of learning that constitute UDL—recognition (knowing *what*), strategy (knowing *how*), and affect (knowing *why*)—and their joint importance for learning to write. We suggest technology tools and teaching methods that in combination support all aspects of the learner.

Universal Design: A Framework for Individualized Learning

CAST's UDL framework posits that learners vary in their needs, styles, and preferences in three specific areas: (1) recognizing patterns, (2) developing strategies for learning, and (3) developing and sustaining engagement. Successful teaching requires the individualization of learning tasks, tools, and content in order to support students in all three areas. To learn to write, students must recognize the patterns of language, must employ expressive skills and strategies, and must persist in these difficult tasks, motivation that usually emerges from having something to say and someone to say it to.

CAST's framework is based in part on recent research in neuroscience and neuropsychology. Evidence in these fields supports the view that three interrelated systems in the brain (a pattern recognition system, a strategic system, and an affective system) work together to enable learning. While the three systems function and interact in roughly the same way for most people, variations in brain structures and functioning lead to highly individual strengths, weaknesses, and approaches to learning within and across systems. Neuroimaging indicates, through individual activity "signatures," that cortex is allocated differently for each person. These differences lead to unique patterns of learning styles and needs, requiring flexible tools and approaches. Tools and approaches that can be adjusted to accommodate differences in the three systems and can provide individually appropriate challenges and supports for different learners are examples of universal design.

Difficulties encountered by students with written language disorders can be understood within this "three brain systems" framework. For example, difficulties with spelling, grammatical conventions, sentence, paragraph, and composition structures (Bain, 1976; Cicci, 1980; Ganschow, 1983; Johnson & Myklebust, 1978; Pompian & Thum, 1988; Roit & McKenzie, 1985; Rubin & Liberman, 1983) fall broadly within the domain of pattern recognition. Difficulties with penmanship, planning, organizing, and attending to audience (Bahr, Nelson, & Van Meter, 1996; Bardine, 1997; Englert & Raphael, 1988; Stillwell & Cermak, 1995; Swanson, 1988) fall broadly within the domain of motor, planning, and strategic skills. Discouragement, poor self-esteem, low expectation of success, and withdrawal of effort from writing tasks (J. W. Chapman & Boersma, 1979; Ellis, 1998; Heyman, 1990; Meyer, 1983b; Raviv & Stone, 1991) fall within the domain of affect and motivation.

To maximize learning opportunities for students with differing abilities, teachers must attend to students' varied skills and needs within each system and, where possible, provide flexible materials, tools, assignments, and supports. Using the UDL framework, we can determine the dimensions along which learning applications must be adjustable in order to meet the needs of a variety of learners within the same classroom. Environments that follow the principles of UDL are adjustable; they provide flexible supports and multiple options in each area to support individual differences between learners. To establish whether a learning environment is universally designed, we evaluate the way information is represented (to adjust to varied recognition systems); the options for teaching strategies and for teaching routine actions (to adjust to varied strategic systems); and the options for content selection, level of challenge, and learning context (to adjust to varied affective systems). Some examples will clarify.

Multiple Representations

Universally designed learning experiences offer varied representations of information to adjust to the recognition needs of all students, including children with learning disabilities, visual or auditory impairments, physical disabilities, and diverse learning preferences. Information that is presented in multiple media (e.g., both printed and spoken text, both image and textual description of the image) or in a medium that allows for easy transformation from one form of representation to another (e.g., digital text transformable to synthetic speech or Braille) allows students to adjust the presentation to suit their own needs. For example, students can change the size, color, or font of digital text to make it easier to see. They can adjust the speed or volume at which text is read aloud by synthetic speech to make it easier to hear.

Multiple Means of Strategy

Universally designed learning experiences can support students' individually different strategic and motor systems by offering varied options for the teaching of writing strategies and varied options for student action (meaning the media used for expression and the motor movements required). For example, universally designed features enable teachers to support strategic approaches to writing, from prewriting through drafting and revision, in different ways for different students.

With software supporting alternative means of action, a student may record spoken ideas digitally and play them back, draw images or diagrams, or enter text. Options for controlling the computer or inputting content can also be adjusted to different motor abilities. Students can use keyboard and mouse, drawing stylus, touch screen, or even a single switch to select among options that are highlighted sequentially on the screen.

Multiple Options for Engagement and Motivation

Universally designed materials accommodate different affective systems, adjusting to students' diverse interests and varied needs for challenge, support, structure, complexity, and novelty. To provide appropriate instruction for all learners, the level of support and the nature of the challenge must be adjustable and able to be individualized. To increase utility and relevance for people from varied social, cultural, ethnic, linguistic, and regional communities, universally designed materials should be "half-full." That is, teachers and students should be able to modify content and activities or add their own (e.g., local images, sounds, text or recorded speech in different languages or dialects). For example, multimedia story programs such as WiggleWorks (1994), a beginning literacy system that combines literature with technology and teacher support, enable learners to replace all or part of an existing story with their own images, text, and sounds.

Recent Advances in Learning Technologies

The application of universal design has become possible in part because of technological innovation, permitting flexibility not imaginable even 10 years ago. Three major trends are most significant:

1. Technology has become more powerful, providing increased speed and connectivity and vast media resources.

2. Technology has become more integrated, providing an array of tools within a single application supporting varied aspects of the writing process.

3. Technology has become more affordable, providing widespread access to powerful writing support tools.

Examples of each of these changes may provide insights about the technological landscape unfolding in our schools and our homes. Please note that our descriptions of features of specific software programs or Web sites in this chapter are not meant as endorsements of those programs or sites.

Increased Power and Connectivity

New, powerful computers and networks bring speed, media capabilities, and connectivity. While early word processors simply "processed words," the capacity to integrate images, sounds, and movies into on-screen compositions, now integral to some word processors, is inherent in the World Wide Web. The Internet provides access to continuously updated information and enables writers to publish work for a potentially huge audience (Leu & Leu, 1997). From elementary school to graduate school, writers are taking advantage of this power in increasing numbers (see Figure 5.1).

Increasingly common are classroom Web sites where student work can be displayed for others in distant places to comment on and see. Further, because the Internet is a multimedia environment, the concept of composition includes not just writing but also expressing ideas through words, images, sounds, videos, and animation. Choice of medium expands the writing toolbox and opens avenues for expression (Meyer, Pisha, & Rose, 1991; Meyer, Rose, & Pisha, 1994). We are just beginning to tap the potential of these technologies for the benefit of learners with written language disorders.

Increased Integration

The word processor of 1991, able to manipulate text and check spelling, seemed powerful then but seems primitive today. Current word processors routinely include an integrated outlining tool, a thesaurus, functional (though imperfect) grammar checking, and the capacity to integrate multimedia into documents. Many current word processors enable users to customize extensively, from formatting menus and toolbars to establishing AutoCorrect preferences, such as replacing *teh* with *the* whenever it is mistyped. Some programs, such as the CAST eReader (1997) and Write:OutLoud (1994), also include text-to-speech (TTS), the capacity to "read" writers' work aloud in synthetic computer voice. TTS provides students with immediate feedback on how their writing sounds when read aloud, an important self-monitoring aid. Speech recognition, another promising technology, enables writers to speak into a microphone and see their words translated into text on the screen. The integration of new tools and increased customizability has vastly improved the capacity of word processing software to support developing writers.

Decreased Cost

Decreasing costs increase access to traditional computers and networks, and to a variety of portable devices that can support writing and organization. A

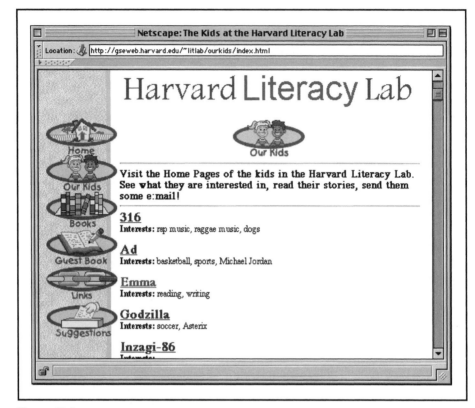

Figure 5.1. Through its Web site, the Harvard Literacy Lab offers children a chance to share their stories with others and invite personal feedback via e-mail. *Note.* Screen shot of Harvard Literacy Lab Web site. Available online: http://gseweb.harvard/edu/~litlab/ourkids/index.html. Copyright by Harvard Literacy Lab. Browser window from Netscape Communicator. Copyright 1999 by Netscape Communications Corp. Used with permission.

prime example is the proliferation of inexpensive electronic notebooks dedicated to word processing with perhaps a few other key functions. Some of these notebooks (e.g., the AlphaSmart) cost less than $250 and can run for weeks on two penlight batteries. Writers can take notes on them in class or at the library, or develop and spell-check drafts of their work, later uploading it to a desktop computer for formatting and printing. The compact size, durability, and low cost of these machines has made them favorites of schools trying to increase the number of computers per student, and of parents who either cannot afford a full-sized laptop for in-class note-taking or worry that their youngsters might either damage or lose such a costly device.

Increased power, connectivity, and integration combined with decreased cost have completely changed the landscape of options and approaches for supporting challenged young writers. Flexibility and customizability are becoming the rule, making it possible to use universal design principles in the classroom to meet the varied recognition, strategic, and affective learning needs of diverse students.

Three Aspects of a Single Complex System

All three brain systems work together in any learning task. The UDL framework is designed to take into account the interconnected nature of these three systems. Though they work together, examining each aspect of UDL separately can help us understand three fundamental aspects of learning and teaching writing, and the ways in which technology can be most helpful in that endeavor.

In the following sections, we highlight examples of technologies and methods tied to each of the three aspects of UDL. We do not present a comprehensive list of available software, nor do we endorse each application we mention. Rather, we highlight examples and offer illustrations of useful features and tools, with the hope that readers will fully evaluate programs and Web sites for themselves and assemble the combination of tools and techniques most effective and applicable to their own classrooms or homes.

A comprehensive set of relevant resources, as well as the full text of this chapter, can be found at the Web site http://www.cast.org.

UDL Part 1: Multiple Means of Supporting the Recognition System in Writing

Introduction to the Recognition System

Skilled writers automatically recognize the patterns of language, from letter shapes or word spellings to formal prose or poetry structures. They understand the conventions of spoken and written language and can easily apply these conventions in their written communication. Reviewing their work, they can evaluate whether they have successfully made their points and whether their work is accurate. The key role of pattern recognition in writing is not as obvious as it is in reading (Meyer & Rose, 1998). Yet the recognition system in the brain plays a crucial role in learning to write and in writing effectively.

Recognition of key language patterns such as letter shapes, spelling conventions, and sentence structures, the province of the posterior brain, is essential to a learner's ability to reproduce these patterns in written expression. To teach pattern recognition, methods and tools should accentuate patterns, offer opportunities to practice applying these patterns, and adjust to individual differences in skills and interests.

Research on the Recognition System in the Brain

The processing necessary to recognize any object is distributed, with color processed in one place, shape in another, orientation and location in still others (Wallis & Bülthoff, 1999). Distributed processing allows the recognition system to operate like an efficient committee, with different brain areas taking on small parts of a task and carrying them out simultaneously. This is the brain's version of what computer scientists call "parallel processing." Its great advantage is speed; a number of systems performing subtasks at the same time (in parallel) is faster than having one system do them one after the other (serially), especially when the work to be done is complex (Cytowic, 1996). At the same time, distributed processing underlies some of the differences in how students learn to recognize patterns. Individuals' varying abilities to identify color, shape, or location mean they face different recognition problems and will respond differently to particular learning materials and teaching techniques.

Distributed, parallel processing of individual elements helps the recognition system to categorize patterns. Indeed, recognition is rooted in classification. Our ability to recognize the letter H depends on understanding the essential elements that define a category we might call "H-ness." Color, size, and whether the symbol is ink on paper, carved wood, or molded plastic are irrelevant. The critical elements are the two generally parallel lines connected by a crossbar somewhere near the middle. The following symbols are not identical, but our understanding of H-ness lets us identify them all as uppercase H.

H   𝓗   ╫

Once thoroughly mastered, categories make future recognition flexible and fast, but learning them is a demanding task, and automatic, accurate recognition requires considerable practice. Recognizing that a particular stimulus fits into an established category is mainly accomplished by the recognition systems. Learning a whole new category, on the other hand, is a whole-brain activity, involving the strategic and affective systems along with the recognition systems (Robin & Holyoak, 1995).

The key role of pattern recognition in writing is illuminated by studying one of the most unusual neurological conditions reported in the literature: alexia without agraphia. Patients with this disorder are completely unable to read (they have alexia) yet they are able to write (they do not have agraphia). Such patients can actually write a sentence, but cannot read their own sentences back (Duffield, de Silva, & Grant, 1994; Erdem & Kansu, 1995). Alexia without agraphia is associated with damage to the posterior cortex, the area of the brain where the recognition system resides. The frontal cortex, where the motor production of written language is generated, is undamaged, enabling a form of writing to take place.

Patients with this syndrome may write, but they do not write well. With a damaged recognition system, their writing is limited to routinized expressions learned before they were injured, and they have limited capacity to generate extended text, or to monitor themselves during or following writing. These findings confirm the critical role played by the recognition system in writing. Recognition is equally essential when students are learning to write and when skilled writers write fluently.

Beginning writers must recognize the conventions of spoken and written language as a part of learning to master them. Learning to form the letter *A* or to write a sentence requires thorough understanding of the target pattern. Accurate knowledge of a pattern is more likely to lead to accurate reproduction of that pattern, though it does not guarantee it. As children are learning, the connection between recognizing and producing must constantly be active. This enables learners to set a goal, write, and evaluate and refine the result. This does not mean that children cannot engage in meaningful communication before mastering the conventional patterns of the language. With appropriate supports, or by using unconventional yet interpretable patterns (such as invented spellings), very young children can communicate effectively in writing. Ultimately, though, mastery of conventions forms the basis for efficient and effective written communication.

Mature, accomplished writers also constantly rely on the recognition system. The brain's recognition mechanisms are critical for all levels of self-monitoring, including evaluating graphemic and syntactic correctness, assessing effectiveness, and determining whether one's purpose has been accomplished. Does the piece conform to the structural requirements of the form (e.g., a letter, a résumé, a persuasive essay)? Does the piece meet the needs of the intended audience? Are the tone and language appropriate? The recognition system is constantly "in the loop" as mature writers write.

For all kinds of neurological reasons, far short of a syndrome such as alexia without agraphia, individuals differ tremendously in their capacity to recognize patterns and to apply that recognition as they write. Problems mastering sound–symbol correspondences, syntactic patterns, paragraph organization, and the structure of various kinds of compositions all can affect both reading and written expression. Awareness of the crucial role of pattern recognition in writing can help teachers support students with diverse recognition problems.

The Recognition System and Writing Instruction

Most teachers find it artificial to make a sharp distinction between the teaching of reading and the teaching of writing. Common sense as well as neurological research confirm that learning to read is deeply intertwined with learning to write, and vice versa. Writers must recognize and be able to apply all of the language patterns that readers use, including letter shapes, sound–symbol correspondences, spelling conventions, sentence structure, syntax, paragraph structures for different types of compositions, and individual writing styles.

Regardless of the level, teachers use both writing and reading lessons to teach these patterns. Structurally, methods for teaching pattern recognition usually fall into one of several general categories: perceptual emphasis, isolating, and grouping according to the target pattern. All of these are designed to heighten attention to and awareness of the nature of the pattern, helping students develop a repertoire of relevant categories.

The most common method of making a pattern easier to recognize is to draw attention to it in context by some kind of perceptual emphasis that makes it stand out from the background. Whether teaching letter formation or letter recognition, a teacher might model the motor movements needed to form the letter as a way of emphasizing its key characteristics. When modeling reading for a group, teachers emphasize language patterns by pointing to words, gesturing, or changing their vocal intonation. Printed materials can emphasize patterns typographically, by using boldface or italic, altering text size or color, or using graphic pointers.

A second method is to isolate examples of the pattern from context, grouping or presenting examples together so that their commonality is more obvious. Grouping spelling words that share a pattern (e.g., the same root, or the same doubling of consonants) is one technique. Another is to group sentences or paragraphs by the same author and contrast them with those of another author. Pattern groups can be presented or students can be asked to sort and generate their own groups by different criteria. Practice at active manipulation of patterns is essential to mastery.

Examples of Technology To Support the Recognition System

Options for teaching writing-related pattern recognition in a digital environment are far more varied, flexible, and customizable than are those in a print-based environment. Through color, animation, and interactivity, computers can help emphasize and isolate patterns, provide opportunities to practice and explore through active manipulation of words and texts, and engage learners' motivation and interest by accommodating individual differences. The flexibility to choose different methods and tools for different students, and the ability to customize the way patterns are presented and practiced, makes the computer an important tool for the universally designed classroom.

Here we address two main categories of pattern: phoneme–letter–word patterns and larger textual patterns. The UDL framework helps us to understand the commonalities between these two categories even though they vary significantly in sophistication. In both, the brain's pattern recognition and categorization systems are at work. The appropriate methods and tools for teaching pattern recognition differ markedly from those best for teaching skills and strategies. Keeping this in mind can help teachers select software and activities appropriate to the task.

A large number of software programs emphasize letter recognition, letter–sound correspondence, phonics, and word recognition (Meyer & Rose, 1998). Varying widely in quality, these programs tend to offer gamelike formats, using color and animation to isolate patterns and direct learners' attention to the critical features that distinguish those patterns. Programs in which letter–sound correspondence, spelling, and word recognition are practiced in a communicative context, with good, relevant feedback, may be most useful for writing, as the practice is occurring in precisely the environment in which the patterns will be applied. For example, in the Read-a-Rhyme exercise in Bailey's Book House (1995), students select from a choice of words to complete a short poem. The feedback—a digitized voice reading back the "new" poem—is directly germane to the reading–writing task and reinforces the learning rather than providing extraneous rewards. Though students are not actually writing, they are composing by selecting words and receiving immediate feedback that demonstrates the results of their work. (A more comprehensive treatment of programs supporting letter- and word-level patterns can be found in Meyer and Rose, 1998, and at http://www.cast.org.)

Perhaps more obviously relevant to writing itself are applications of computers to teaching larger textual patterns such as story grammars, essay structures, or letter-writing formats. Computers are useful for highlighting textual patterns, particularly through the use of templates. Holding constant the key structural components of a pattern and enabling students to manipulate the content provides a highly interactive lesson in pattern recognition. Some examples will illustrate.

The Amazing Writing Machine

The Amazing Writing Machine (1994) is designed to foster writing in elementary school children. It is divided into five writing projects: Essay, Letter, Story, Poem, and Journal. Each project can be completed in one of two modes. In the Write mode, the student creates the project completely "from scratch." The other, called the Spin mode, aids the recognition system by providing a prewritten composition that includes blank sections in which students select from a group of words or phrases to complete a sentence. For example, the Spin Journal begins, "My day began when I woke up _____." The student can either pick a given word or phrase (e.g., *early, late*) or type one in. This format helps students learn to recognize the features that are important in each of the writing project formats (see Figure 5.2). Pictures are also included that can be colored to illustrate the project. For teachers who may feel constrained by the tight

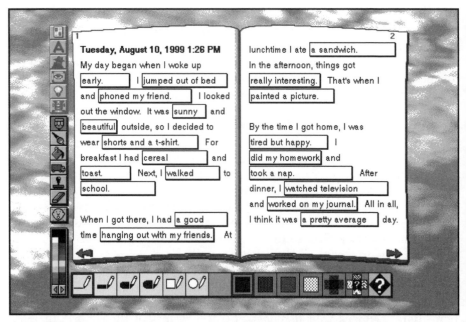

Figure 5.2. The Spin mode of the Amazing Writing Machine program gives students a prewritten composition with blanks. *Note.* Screen shot of Amazing Writing Machine. Copyright 1994 by Brøderbund. Used with permission.

structure of this program, similar effects can be created in a regular word processor with a "lock" or "protect" text feature, enabling teachers to create their own documents in which only selected sections can be edited.

Microsoft Word

Microsoft Word (1998) offers a variety of formats and templates to support writers as they generate text. For example, the Letter Wizard provides help with the physical layout of the page, showing visually where letter parts should be placed and how paragraphs should be structured for different styles of letter (see Figure 5.3). Further, writers can fill in labeled spaces for salutation, recipient's name, sender's name and address, and so on, and items will automatically be placed in the correct locations on screen. Microsoft Word offers wizards for many written formats including agendas, brochures, résumés, newsletters, press releases, and even a "thesis template." In some cases, the program includes actual samples which serve as models of completed compositions. Many other word processors have similar features; readers should evaluate a variety of programs to determine which one best suits their and their students' needs.

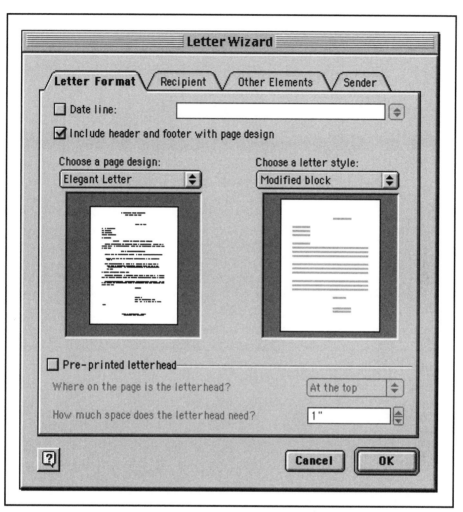

Figure 5.3. The Microsoft Word Letter Wizard offers help with the physical layout of the page. *Note.* Screen shot from Microsoft Word 98. Copyright 1983–1998 by Microsoft Corp. All rights reserved. Used with permission.

HyperStudio

Syntactical structures can be improvised and practiced using a regular word processor or, for young writers, a multimedia program like HyperStudio (1994) with the capacity for drawing, speech, and sound. Teachers can place text or poem structures on successive screens and invite students to modify text, images, and sounds to create class books or group multimedia projects.

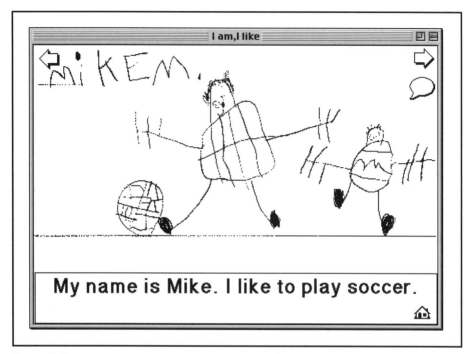

Figure 5.4. "I am I like" Hypercard stack. Young writers can practice improvised syntactical structures with multimedia programs.

With some text structures kept constant and selective elements available for modification, students grasp textual patterns by working actively with them (see Figure 5.4).

Organizer and outliner programs are also helpful for teaching textual structures. These programs help make organizational and hierarchical relationships explicit for students who may not pick them up easily. Some outliner and visual organizer programs, such as Inspiration, display textual content graphically in "bubble" maps. Teachers can create models, or templates, for the structures of written expression. Examples range from the prototypical paragraph with its topic sentence and several supporting sentences to the structure of a Greek myth, including a hero, a villain, a struggle, and a resolution, in idea map form. The latter can include bubbles labeled according to the structure, but left empty for students to fill. This provides students with a model for the structure of the writing, but leaves them free to generate their own ideas within that structure. A word of caution, however, on the flexibility of programs such as Inspiration: Some students become so enamored of all of the formatting options that they "play" much of the time and spend little time on serious work.

Awareness of the recognition system's role in writing can help teachers be more deliberate in their selection of tools, tasks, and supports, and technology provides a powerful ally for teaching writing-related pattern recognition, from letter shapes to author's style. With technology tools, assignments, practice content, and feedback can be customized for different learners, making universally designed pattern recognition activities feasible in classrooms of students with widely varied learning needs.

UDL Part 2: Multiple Means of Supporting the Strategic System in Writing

Introduction to the Strategic System

When the strategic system is working efficiently, a student is able to determine the purpose or goal of a written assignment, organize the relevant information, determine an appropriate structure, and evaluate the results. At the same time, the mechanics of writing flow automatically; conscious energy is not diverted to what needs to be routine. The strategic system is responsible both for the deliberate planning of complex actions and for routine actions that occur automatically, and mostly not consciously. Both are essential components of learning to write.

The high-level strategic skills needed for written expression—developing a plan that will meet a goal, organizing information to implement the plan, and monitoring the work as it progresses—require the involvement of the strategic system, located in the anterior (frontal) part of the brain. This region also has primary responsibility for routine output skills in writing, from letter formation or touch typing to producing well-structured sentences. The principles of UDL, supported by research on the brain, tie together the continuum of skills that fall under the strategic system and help us understand that teaching this continuum requires a different approach than does teaching pattern recognition. Optimal skill instruction includes the key elements of apprenticeship: models of expert performance, scaffolded practice in a meaningful context, ongoing feedback on performance, and opportunities to demonstrate progress.

In this section, we address the teaching of strategic writing skills and the teaching of routine writing actions separately, though both fall broadly within the strategic segment of UDL, and both call for an apprenticeship model of teaching.

Research on the Brain's Strategic System

The anterior portions of the frontal lobes are essential in developing strategies and plans for reaching a goal, particularly in situations in which there is no clear path to take. The functions of the strategic system in high-level planning can be divided into four stages.

First, this system plays a critical role in "sizing up" a situation and determining a plan that will be effective (Elfgren & Risberg, 1998; Gershberg & Shimamura, 1995; Goel, Grafman, Tajik, Gana, & Danto, 1997). In order to work effectively, the strategic system must be able to organize, categorize, manipulate, and determine the importance of information about the problem at hand (Osherson et al., 1998).

The second part of the planning process involves modeling or visualizing the plan and its potential results before actually initiating any action. In this way, the adequacy and completeness of the plan, as well as the time it will take and its likely effectiveness, can be judged and the plan can be modified before it is begun (Goel & Grafman, 1995; Goel et al., 1997).

Third, the strategic system monitors the plan as it is being implemented. While the plan is carried out, the strategic system receives information from both the environment and other areas of the brain (e.g., the motor and affective systems) about how well it is working. This information helps determine whether each step in the plan has been adequately completed (Goel et al., 1997). This information can then be used to revise the plan or to shift strategies during its implementation (Blakemore, Rees, & Frith, 1998; Jeannerod, 1997).

Finally, after a plan has been carried out, the strategic system determines how well the goal has been met. The knowledge of the results also is incorporated for use in future planning (Jeannerod, 1997).

Strategy and Writing Instruction

Understanding individual differences in strategic skills can help teachers be more effective in teaching the now-traditional elements of process writing, including three broad phases: prewriting, drafting, and revising. Prewriting is the planning phase. Drafting and revising are the phases in which students monitor and evaluate their own work relative to the purpose or goal of the writing (Hallenbeck, 1995).

Many students with learning difficulties have trouble at the beginning stages of planning or strategizing. They may plunge into a task without having all the information needed or they may approach the task in a random fashion (Bardine, 1997; MacArthur, 1996). Students with problems at this level may write on subjects that are totally unrelated to the topic. Others may understand the purpose for writing but have trouble organizing and structuring information so that it can be used for a specific purpose, such as telling a story or supporting a point of view (Zipprich, 1995).

Students who have problems with the modeling phase of strategic planning do not think through an assignment. Often they merely plan for it in the way they have approached previous assignments, not seeing aspects unique to the current situation. They cannot anticipate the possible shortcomings or stumbling blocks inherent in their plans (Butler, 1995). Additionally, they do not have a clear sense of how much time their plan will take. They either allow too much time or (more frequently) develop a large-scale plan that cannot be accomplished adequately in the time allotted.

Some students can devise a plan for solving a problem or completing an assignment but are unaware of points during the implementation when the plan needs to be modified. They develop a plan that will work "in theory," but do not monitor effectively enough to notice when conditions change and an additional step or another approach is needed (Meltzer, 1991). When writing, students may not incorporate new information into an argument. They may not see that changing the order of two paragraphs would enhance an argument.

Alternately, some students may deviate from a plan and not be aware that they have done so. Other stimuli in the environment may attract their attention, and soon they are going off in a different direction. In addition, they may have trouble allowing sufficient time for each step of the plan. Either they become bogged down in a fact-finding/research phase and never get to the actual writing of the paper or, more frequently, they leave the entire project until the very last moment or forget to even begin it until other students are handing in their work during class.

Finally, students may not be aware that what they have produced does not meet the requirements of an assignment. Certainly, an inadequate plan and ineffective monitoring will result in less than optimal results. Students may not have the skills to judge the quality of their work or to analyze how effectively it meets the goals that were established initially. Without this reflective analysis, students cannot revise the current assignment (Hallenbeck, 1995; Wong, Butler, Ficzere, & Kuperis, 1996).

Examples of Technology to Support Strategy

Students who have trouble with higher level strategic skills benefit from supports for the generation, organization, and elaboration of ideas for writing. The UDL approach can help teachers select technology tools that support the elements of apprenticeship (modeling, supported practice, individual feedback, and opportunities to demonstrate mastery) and allow individualization to accommodate learners' varied strategic strengths and weaknesses. Some examples illustrate.

Writer's Solution: Writing Lab

Writer's Solution: Writing Lab (1997) is an example of a program that models the writing process as a whole. It divides the process into four stages: prewriting, drafting, revising, and presenting. Each step includes an explanation of what will be done and why it is important; several different activities to help make the actions explicit; and an example of what a product looks like at that stage in the process. It also includes a map, viewable at any time, that shows all of the stages of the process, along with the steps in each stage. This helps students to develop the internal model of where a plan is leading (see Figures 5.5 and 5.6).

Writer's Helper

Another tool offering supported practice for the strategic writing process is Writer's Helper (1997). Working with word processors and adding supports

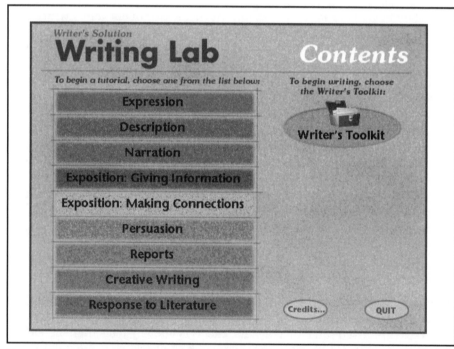

Figure 5.5. Writer's Solution choice screen. An example of a program that models the writing process as a whole. *Note.* Screen shot adapted from Writer's Solution: Writing Lab for Macintosh. Copyright 1997 by Prentice Hall. Used with permission.

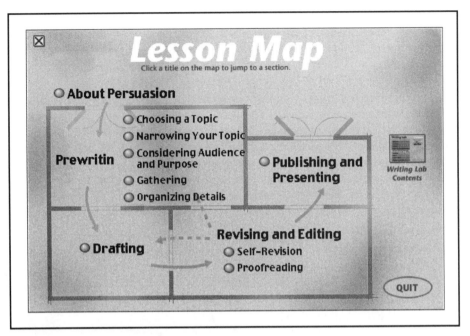

Figure 5.6. Writer's Solution Lesson Map. A visual map of the writing process can help students develop an internal model. *Note.* Screen shot adapted from Writer's Solution: Writing Lab for Macintosh. Copyright 1997 by Prentice Hall. Used with permission.

for planning, writing, and editing, Writer's Helper includes help with each step and generates a "notebook" with both the prompts and the student's responses. Work can then be exported to a word processor for editing and revising. The flexibility of this tool—offering a range of supports from structured to open-ended—is an example of a universally designed feature that supports customized approaches for students with a variety of learning styles.

Researchpaper.com

Researchpaper.com, a Web site (http://www.researchpaper.com), also supports practice by making self-monitoring explicit. The site contains an Idea Directory that provides help in generating ideas for a paper (prewriting stage) and a Writing Center, where a student can find instructions and checklists for the actual steps in writing, including help with both composition and mechanics. Relevant feedback, another key element of apprenticeship, can be found in Research Central, an area that supports discussion between students and links to experts that can help guide on-line research. An example of well-applied connectivity, this feature illustrates how technology can be an avenue for individual feedback that teachers may not be able to personally provide for each student (see Figure 5.7).

Inspiration

Idea organizing and visual mapping are techniques that can be implemented on or off the computer. The capacity to create "half-full" templates for content and structure, however, make technology-based idea mapping ideal for creating universally designed environments. Inspiration (1997), an outliner and visual organizer, provides alternative ways of representing relationships between ideas and therefore accommodates different learners' needs. The subject of considerable research attention (Anderson-Inman & Horney, 1996–1997; Anderson-Inman, Knox-Quinn, & Horney, 1996; Anderson-Inman, Redekopp, & Adams, 1992;

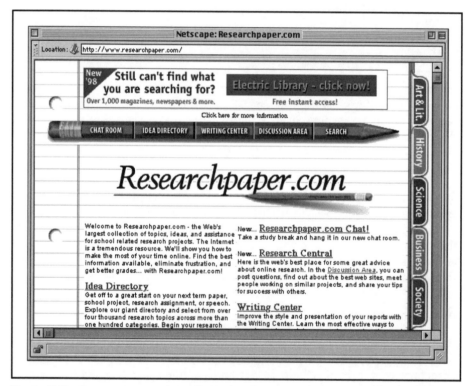

Figure 5.7. Researchpaper.com Web site. Web sites support discussion between students about their ideas for research and writing. *Note.* Screen shot of Researchpaper.com. Available online: http://www.researchpaper.com. Copyright by Infonautics Corp. Used with permission. Browser window from Netscape Communicator. Copyright 1999 by Netscape Communications Corp. Used with permission.

Anderson-Inman & Zeitz, 1993, 1994), Inspiration helps writers generate either traditionally structured hierarchical outlines or graphical idea maps that represent relationships between ideas through geometric shapes, spatial orientation, and connecting lines. In either mode, this program supports brainstorming by making it easy to move ideas around on the computer screen and to experiment with different arrangements or sequences. When key ideas are arranged in an organized form, students can better see gaps in their writing plan and move to fill them (see Figures 5.8 and 5.9).

Software with Text-to-Speech Feature

Feedback, a key feature of apprenticeship and one that is difficult for teachers to provide individually, can be generated with a powerful technology feature,

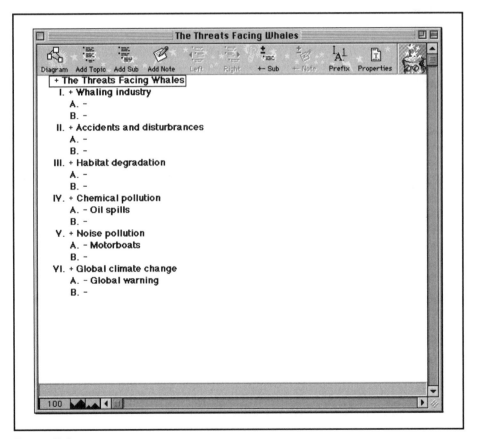

Figure 5.8. Inspiration document outline view. Software like Inspiration can help with the organization of ideas for writing. *Note*. Screen shot from Inspiration. Copyright 1988–1994 by Inspiration software. Used with permission.

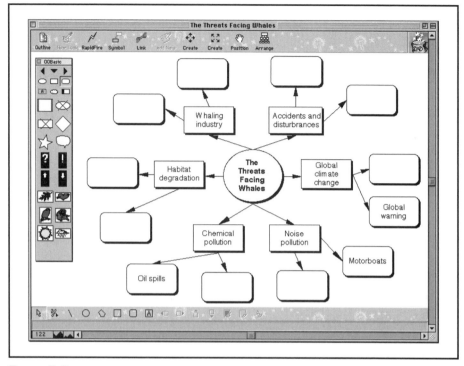

Figure 5.9. Inspiration document diagram view (slightly reduced to fit page, image may be degraded). With Inspiration, options for textual or graphical formatting accommodate learner preferences. *Note.* Screen shot from Inspiration. Copyright 1988–1994 by Inspiration software. Used with permission.

text-to-speech (TTS), the feature that allows the computer to read back any written text in a synthesized computer voice. TTS is deceptively simple, yet it helps students monitor and evaluate their work independently. Several programs (e.g., IntelliTalk, 1993; Write:OutLoud, 1994; and CAST eReader, 1997) incorporate TTS, which can be set to read each letter, each word, or each sentence as it is typed, or only on request after writing (see Figure 5.10).

With TTS, writers can hear their own work read aloud, as others might hear it. This feedback is extremely useful in helping writers with learning disabilities check for errors in formulation, such as incomplete sentences or misspelled words, omitted or duplicated words, or words inadvertently selected from a list presented by a spell checker (MacArthur, 1998). TTS can also help students monitor the match between their goals and their completed compositions, or between the assignment and the outcome. Thus TTS supports the monitoring of both writing strategies and routine actions.

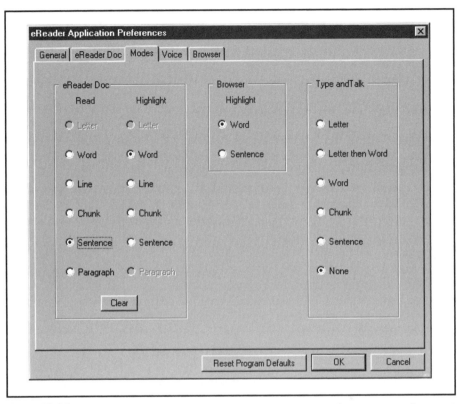

Figure 5.10. CAST eReader. Text-to-speech programs can be set to read text at the level most helpful to the individual. *Note*. Screen shot from CAST eReader. Copyright 1995–1997, 1999 by CAST. Used with permission.

Research on Routine Actions in the Brain

Most actions that we produce during the course of the day are routine or automatic; they make little or no demand on our conscious attention. However, these routine actions are essential for our ability to function day to day (D. Chapman, 1991). Control of these well-practiced actions appears to be located primarily in the more posterior areas of the frontal lobes (Karni et al., 1998; Petersen, van Mier, Fiez, & Raichle, 1998; Posner & Raichle, 1994). There is some evidence that prefrontal regions are involved in monitoring routine actions for errors. Patients with prefrontal lesions have demonstrated a variety of difficulties, including perseverating on one action (i.e., repeating it), leaving out steps or changing the sequence of actions, and difficulty suppressing incorrect responses (Burgess & Shallice, 1996; Cooper & Shallice, 1997).

The development of routine actions requires extensive practice to make them automatic. When this is achieved, the anterior frontal regions of the brain are involved only in monitoring for errors, not in the actual execution of the action.

Routine Actions and Writing Instruction

All students occasionally make errors in actions that they produce automatically. But many students with learning disabilities have particular difficulty in monitoring their routine actions and catching and correcting their mistakes. Because these actions do not take much conscious effort, students may be more likely to leave out or mix up steps, perseverate an action, or give incorrect responses, without being aware of their errors. Competent writers are able to generate grammatically correct sentences and transform them into written language on an automatic level (MacArthur, 1996). Students with written language disorders may lack automaticity in the mechanics of written production (including letter formation and spelling problems), in sentence formulation, or in other aspects of writing demanding rapid execution of patterned activity. The need to consciously attend to skills that should be automatic limits a student's ability to engage in the higher order cognitive activities needed for effective writing (MacArthur, 1998; Martin & Manno, 1995).

Guided practice and relevant feedback, both key parts of apprenticeship learning, figure importantly in routinizing the motor and strategic actions necessary for writing. Though traditional methods such as worksheets and customized approaches such as allowing students to bypass the routine (e.g., dictating to a teacher instead of handwriting) can be implemented without a computer, technology tools offer more flexible, powerful means both to scaffold (or support) weak areas and to learn the necessary routines. The best of these tools can be customized, making them important parts of a universally designed environment.

Examples of Technology To Support the Strategic System in Routine Actions

The most obvious routine action in written production is handwriting. Until a child can form letters efficiently and automatically, much of the conscious effort in writing will be directed toward this task, rather than toward the larger goal of written expression.

While those with significant motor disabilities have difficulty with handwriting (and may never become functional writers), others with less obvious motor deficits also find handwriting difficult. Their problem may be due to poor fine motor control, which affects the complex distal finger movements needed to manipulate a pencil; due to difficulty remembering what the letters look like; or due to a more specific difficulty in translating the image of a letter into a motor output (Cermak, 1991; Stillwell & Cermak, 1995; Ziviani, 1995). Additionally, some children are able to write quickly and automatically, but their writing is so poor that it can be read only by those who are familiar with it. Improving legibility comes at the cost of automaticity.

Word Processing and Keyboarding Programs

If handwriting is not a routine action, whether because of frank or subtle deficits, then the most common alternative is computer word processing. Word processing is now used by most students for some, if not all, written assignments, and it is rapidly becoming the primary method of formal written production in schools. Word processing enables students to produce assignments that are both legible and neat, and it is a great help to children whose handwriting cannot be read easily. Ease of revising and editing are also among its benefits.

Word processing requires that students learn to keyboard, a new skill that at first seems easier to acquire than handwriting skills, especially for children with fine motor problems and difficulties learning routine actions. Pisha (1993) studied keyboarding skill acquisition in 92 fourth-, fifth-, and sixth-graders, 40% of whom had identified mild special needs (but no severe motor deficits). Speed of handwriting was predictive of the speed of keyboarding skill acquisition; students with special needs were slower at keyboarding initially and acquired keyboarding skills more slowly than others, but both groups learned faster when they worked with a keyboarding tutorial program.

The motor component in keyboarding requires less complex movements than does handwriting, but does carry some challenges. Keyboarding requires a good sense of spatial position of the fingers. Additionally, children must learn a spatial layout for the letters of the alphabet that does not correspond to the order in which they are typically seen. Keyboarding requires a shifting of attention between the keyboard and the screen, particularly during learning. As with any skill that needs to become routine, keyboarding requires a great deal of practice. Key features in high-quality keyboarding programs include an on-screen spatial representation of finger positions; a logical sequence of keys taught in ascending complexity; clear presentation of the target letters; mastery of each level required before proceeding to the next level; frequent feedback about progress including accuracy and speed; and engaging activities that are fun, especially for younger children. Programs such as Mavis Beacon Teaches Typing (1999) and Type to Learn (1992) provide these elements (see Figure 5.11).

Many other programs are available through computer stores and catalogs. If a child is learning keyboarding because of difficulty with fine motor

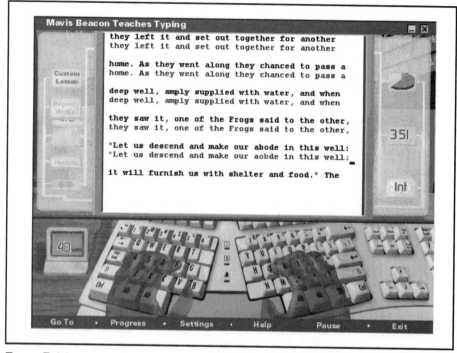

Figure 5.11. Mavis Beacon. Well-designed keyboarding programs provide frequent feedback. *Note.* Screen shot from Mavis Beacon Teaches Typing (Ver. 10, Deluxe). Copyright 1988, 1992 by Brøderbund. Used with permission.

skills, it is important to use a program that does not emphasize speed over accuracy. The best programs include the option to turn features (such as time) on and off. Word processors with speech synthesis built in (e.g., My Words, 1993; CAST eReader, 1997; Write:OutLoud, 1994) can also be used to help children learn to type by setting them to speak the letters as they are typed, thus providing immediate feedback.

Abbreviation Expansion and Word Prediction Software Features

Typing programs help students build automaticity, and using a word processor supports routine writing at the level of letter entry. But the current writing toolbox provides varied support for higher level routine actions as well. Students with writing difficulties often misspell common words and phrases that they need to use frequently. Two features found in many word processors—abbreviation expansion and word prediction—can speed text entry and improve accuracy. With abbreviation expansion, the user types a predetermined abbreviation for a word or phrase and the abbreviation is automati-

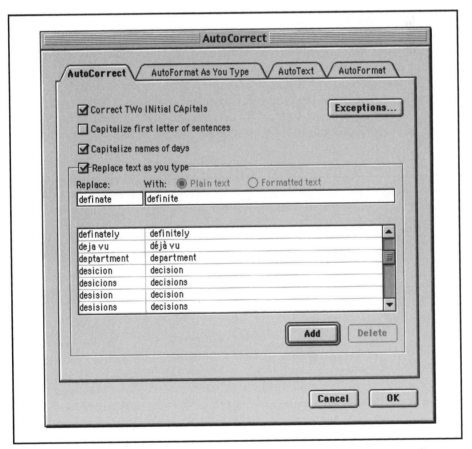

cally expanded (or typed on screen) into the complete word or phrase. The AutoCorrect feature in Microsoft Word serves this function. In addition to its more usual application of correcting common typing errors, users can enter abbreviations for words or phrases. When the abbreviation is typed, Microsoft Word will automatically expand it to the full word or phrase (see Figure 5.12).

AutoCorrect exemplifies universal design in that it is customizable and operates only if the writer chooses to use it. A teacher or parent can work with a student to choose words and phrases and select their abbreviations to facilitate written expression. AutoCorrect can also be used to correct common misspellings or typing errors as the student is writing. The learning context,

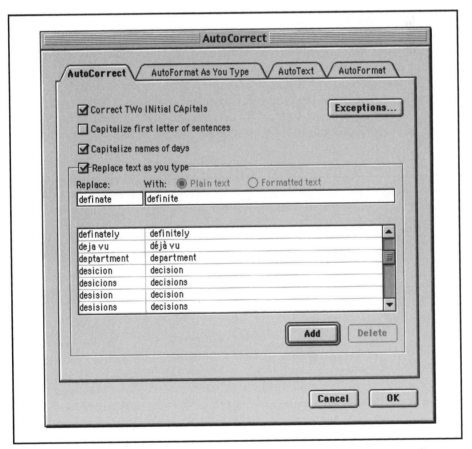

Figure 5.12. Microsoft Word AutoCorrect. AutoCorrect can be set up to fix commonly misspelled or mistyped words. *Note.* Screen shot from Microsoft Word 98. Copyright 1983–1998 by Microsoft Corp. All rights reserved. Used with permission.

however, is important. If the purpose of a writing session is to help the student to learn to spell correctly, AutoCorrect should be turned off. If the purpose is to produce an accurately spelled document for a content-area assignment, AutoCorrect should be turned on.

Word prediction also supports writers with automatic production difficulties. Drawing on a stored set of words, programs with word prediction generate suggested options for completing words during text entry. When the first letter is typed, the program presents a list of possible words beginning with that letter, based on both spelling and syntax. As each additional letter is typed, the list is refined. When the intended word appears in the list, the user selects it, by clicking on it or typing its number, and the program inserts the word into the document. Mechanisms for presenting and inserting words range from a scrolling word list in a separate window (My Words) to a pop-up of frequently used words or phrases that can be inserted by pressing the return key (Microsoft Word).

Co:Writer (1993) functions as a separate text-entry window with any word processor. When a sentence is completed, it is automatically placed into the word processor document (see Figure 5.13).

Co:Writer also provides text-to-speech support and uses a form of artificial intelligence to build the frequency lists for prediction. That is, words the writer actually types most frequently become the first on the list in the prediction window. This can be a plus or a minus, as students with writing diffi-

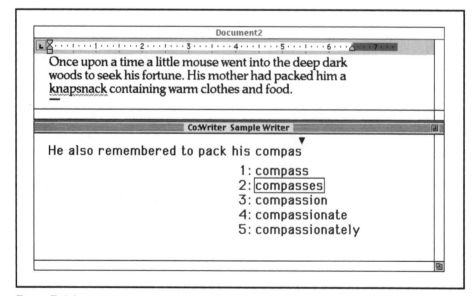

Figure 5.13. Co:Writer can help build students' self-monitoring skills. *Note.* Screen shot from Co:Writer. Copyright 1992 by Don Johnson, Inc. Used with permission.

culties often misspell a word the same way multiple times. Thus an incorrectly spelled word could top the frequency list. Fortunately, it is possible to clear and edit the list, an exercise that could be useful in helping to build students' self-monitoring skills if done collaboratively.

Word prediction lowers the number of keystrokes, and supports children with severe spelling problems, as frequently only the first few letters of a word need be typed (MacArthur, 1998). Studies are also suggesting that word prediction may actually improve writing and spelling accuracy for students with learning disabilities. In a study on the effects of word processing with word prediction on the writing accuracy of handwritten response journals among a small sample of students with learning disabilities, MacArthur found that four out of five students improved their writing legibility and spelling accuracy. Lewis, Graves, Ashton, and Kieley (1998) compared a group of students with learning disabilities and a control group using a variety of text-entry methods including word processors with word prediction. Handwriting was the fastest overall means of text entry, followed by word processing with word prediction. All technology groups improved writing and spelling accuracy, and the gap between writers with and without learning disabilities narrowed on the dimension of text accuracy.

These findings suggest that word prediction has significant promise as an important writing scaffold for students with learning disabilities, and may even improve their routine skills. Because it interrupts the flow of typing, and therefore can be frustrating for students wishing to keep up with the flow of their ideas, it may be helpful to teach word prediction as a skill in its own right. Research is needed to clarify whether word prediction is most effectively taught when students are learning keyboarding or after keyboarding skills are automatized.

Speech Recognition Software

Speech recognition, another new technology supporting text entry, is becoming increasingly available, affordable, and effective. It allows users to sidestep both handwriting and keyboarding and enter text into a computer by speaking into a microphone. The computer then digitizes the voice and compares it to stored information, producing on-screen text of what the user has said. In essence, speech recognition takes dictation from the writer. This long-awaited capability is now available in a form that, while still imperfect, is increasingly usable and is improving rapidly. Speech recognition software such as ViaVoice (1998), OutSPOKEN (1992), and Naturally Speaking (1997) are compatible with desktop computers and are now available for under $200.

To use speech recognition, writers must first train the system to recognize their voices by speaking controlled texts into the microphone. The machine matches the reader's voice to its stored list and uses the match as the basis of subsequent recognition. The training requirement, in some cases demanding more than an hour of careful reading, is a limitation of speech recognition. Some students lack the patience or the reading skills to complete the training. Dividing training into shorter time periods and coaching students on the required reading passages can help with this. Another concern with speech recognition is the somewhat cumbersome procedure for correcting errors made by the computer. Finding and correcting these errors is another skill set that students must automatize for optimal use of the system. The most promising solution to problems with training and accuracy is continued advances in technology itself, which appear to be rapid and ongoing.

Despite the training and correction obstacles, teachers and students are beginning to use speech recognition software. In addition to the obvious elimination of the need to hand write or to keyboard, this technology also provides powerful support in the spelling area; if the word is recognized accurately, the computer always selects the correct spelling. Thus, writers can represent their ideas in one medium, speech, and have the computer convert it into another, text. Early research at both elementary and postsecondary levels suggests that speech recognition holds promise for students with written language disorders (Higgins & Raskind, 1995; Wetzel, 1996).

UDL Part 3: Multiple Means of Supporting the Affective System in Writing

Introduction to the Affective System

Communication is the essence of writing. Creating a narrative, writing a letter or an e-mail, keeping a journal, or noting reactions to what one has read all imply a dialogue between the writer and a reader, even if the reader is oneself. Students fully engaged in writing find themselves deeply immersed in an exchange, with further efforts fueled by responses themselves evoked by a give-and-take of ideas.

The affective system fuels the motivation to write, the ability to adopt different styles to suit different purposes, the confidence to persist, and the love of communication. Fostering engagement in writing requires the ability to adjust content, vary the level of challenge, provide appropriate supports, offer timely feedback, and provide a number of contexts for writing so that students with different interests, abilities, and preferences can all find experiences that have strong appeal.

Students may come to love writing for many different reasons. Writing may give them an opportunity to exercise and extend an area of competence; they may relish stories and be inspired to write by what they read; they may use writing to build relationships with friends or with mentors; or writing may be the vehicle through which they clarify their thinking or express their emotions. Because learning to write is a long and complex process, especially for students with language processing disorders, engaging students in writing is critical to the teacher's success.

Research on the Affective System in the Brain

Although teachers have long known the importance of motivation and enthusiasm, affective aspects of the brain and learning have only recently become the subject of intensive research (Damasio, 1994; D'Arcangelo, 1998; Jensen, 1998; LeDoux, 1996). Increasingly, evidence suggests that the affective system plays a critical role in students' ability to learn (Howard, 1994; Meyer & Rose, 1998; Sylvester, 1998; Wolfe & Brandt, 1998). Both the recognition and the strategic systems' functioning is intimately tied to the attitudes and emotions generated by the affective system (Wolfe & Brandt, 1998). Affective factors underlie students' ability to set priorities, to focus attention, to select among competing stimuli and competing possibilities for action, and, ultimately, to persist, practice, and master material and skills.

The affective system exerts physiological influences on cognitive functions. For instance, subsystems of the affective system turn information about our blood sugar levels into feelings about food. When blood sugar is low, our desire for food increases. We are motivated to eat, and the craving for food may make it difficult to concentrate on anything else. The affective system determines whether we seek food, rest, safety, and other fundamental necessities. It also influences our interest in novelty, challenge, particular subjects, and different kinds of learning contexts (Ellis, 1998; Howard, 1994; Morrison & Cosden, 1997). We are drawn to novelty when we feel understimulated; when we are overwhelmed with stimulation, we avoid novelty (Meyer & Rose, 1998).

The affective system regulates immediate perceptions and actions, and also builds habitual responses to tasks and circumstances. These "habits of mind" (the routines of the affective system) lead us to associate feelings with certain kinds of experiences, even though a current experience may not legitimately evoke such feelings. The power of these associations was shown clearly in an experiment with an amnesiac patient, who learned and remembered feelings about a person even with no conscious recognition of the person's face or name (LeDoux, 1996). We all have emotional memories associated with events no longer conscious. We seek experiences associated with positive feelings and avoid those associated with pain or humiliation. These observations are consistent with case studies and research reports delineating complex emotional concomitants of learning disability, where failure and frustration may become associated with learning experiences (Athey, 1976; Butkowsky & Willows, 1980; Heyman, 1990; Huntington & Bender, 1993; Meyer, 1983b; Pullis, 1988; Raviv & Stone, 1991; Rourke & Fisk, 1981).

One important facet of engagement is an optimal level of challenge, one that draws attention and interest, and is not beyond reach. Decades ago, Vygotsky (1962) introduced the concept of the "zone of proximal development" (ZPD) or the "distance between the child's actual development level . . . and the child's level of potential development" (Englert, Rozendal, & Mariage, 1994, p. 187) achievable with support from a teacher or peer. When challenge is at precisely the right level for a student, the task is just within reach with support. The appropriate level of challenge can be deeply engaging for learners, a state Csikszentmihályi (1997) called "flow."

> Flow tends to occur when a person's skills are fully involved in overcoming a challenge that is just about manageable. . . . When goals are clear, feedback relevant, and challenges and skills are in balance, attention becomes ordered and fully invested. Because of the total demand on psychic energy, a person in flow is completely focused. (Csikszentmihályi, 1997, pp. 30–31)

Neuropharmacological evidence supports the concept of an optimal level of challenge. Studies in which subjects were overchallenged showed overproduction of neurotransmitters, impeding learning by increasing stress (Koob, Cole, Swerdlow, & leMoal, 1990; LeDoux, 1996). Studies in which subjects were underchallenged showed underproduction of neurotransmitters, engendering apathy (Schultz, Dayan, & Montague, 1997; Wolfe & Brandt, 1998).

As we learn more about the workings of the affective system in the brain, we can approach teaching and technology with a more sophisticated sense of what each student needs.

The Affective System and Writing Instruction

> It is as if we are possessed by a passion for reason, a drive that originates in the brain core, permeates other levels of the nervous system, and emerges as either feelings or nonconscious biases to guide decision making. Reason . . . is probably constructed on this inherent drive by a process which resembles the mastering of a skill or craft. Remove the drive, and you will not acquire the mastery. But having the drive does not automatically make you a master. (Damasio, 1994, p. 144)

How can teachers and developers of writing curricula and technology use insights about the affective system to create optimal learning experiences that support student engagement at all levels of skill? In their article relating brain research to instruction, Tomlinson and Kalbfleisch (1998) called for "differentiated classrooms [which are] emotionally safe for learning, [provide] appropriate levels of challenge [for each student, and provide opportunities for] each brain [to] make its own meaning of ideas and skills" (p. 54). The authors described characteristics of such a classroom, which include great flexibility and individualization of learning contexts, assignments, presentation of ideas, expressive media, and levels of challenge. They did not, however, address the difficulty faced by a single teacher or team of teachers in providing such complex layers of individualization, nor did they suggest tools and techniques that could make it possible.

Just as subject matter interest is highly individual, so is the ideal context for motivating writing. Some students are most productive and happy working face-to-face with a teacher or peer, while others are highly engaged by e-mail exchanges. Where classrooms themselves used to be the only viable learning context, the World Wide Web makes it possible to expand the geographical context or shift the time and place of working, finding support, and exchanging feedback. University professors as well as elementary teachers are increasingly able to offer online office hours to review work and offer suggestions via e-mail and to post resources and supports on Web sites accessible to students 24 hours a day. This flexibility can help students find the time, place, and circumstances most beneficial for them.

Examples of Technology To Support the Affective System

The adjustability necessary to engage students with varied skills, needs, styles, and interests can, in our view, be provided only through the use of technology in support of universal design. The flexibility inherent in digital media, when employed to provide customizable options in software, and the almost limitless possibilities offered by the World Wide Web, support our ability to individualize the teaching and learning of writing.

Drawing upon research in neuropsychology, education, and psychology, we find five key dimensions of instruction for which the adjustability of technology can be pivotal in engaging students in learning to write. These dimensions are:

1. Adjustable level of challenge

2. Varied supports

3. Timely and relevant feedback

4. Material that sparks personal interest

5. Variable learning contexts

Enthusiastic writers work at an appropriate level of challenge; find the supports they need; get prompt, relevant feedback; write on subjects that are personally relevant and interesting; and find a context for writing that excites their interest.

One might argue that because learning to write is especially difficult for students with learning disabilities, and because it takes such a long time, supporting engagement for these students is particularly critical (Heyman, 1990; Meyer, 1983a; White, Moffitt, & Silva, 1992). In addressing the key affective dimensions and how to support them, we assume a supportive learning environment using meaningful writing tasks within a framework of process writing (Englert et al., 1994; MacArthur, 1996; Palincsar & Klenk, 1992).

Equally critical are "universally designed assignments," that are themselves customized to fulfill the particular purpose a teacher has in mind and to adjust to the affective needs of different students. Teachers who clearly define the purpose of their assignments can individualize students' means for completing the work, enabling them, for example, to select a medium of expression that suits their own style and preference.

For example, if the teaching goal is to help students learn to create narratives, teachers can offer varied media options including sequences of images, sounds, words, animations, or a combination of media. Students who have difficulty with text, but who love to draw or work with sound, can become engaged in the assignment via their medium of choice. If, however, the goal is to create textual narratives, the ultimate expressive medium must be text, but scaffolds to support text generation and monitoring (such as word prediction or voice recognition) can be differentially provided to adjust to individual skill levels. In both cases, the teaching goal dictates the kinds of flexibility that are appropriate, and the principles of universal design for learning can be applied.

Software with Adjustable Levels of Challenge

In his studies into the enormous appeal of computer games, Malone (1981, 1984) identified incrementally adjustable challenge levels as critical factors. The most successful games, such as Lode Runner or Tetris, meet players at their level of competence and then induce them to move beyond it, in manageable steps. In the realm of writing instruction, it would be rare to encounter a learning task as highly constrained and structured as those found in computer games. Thus finding and teaching to students' ZPDs requires a willingness to provide less highly constrained experiences that meet each student at the edge of his or her competence and provide support for moving ahead.

Multimedia composing tools such as HyperStudio (1994) or WiggleWorks (1994) offer teachers the opportunity to present writing tasks with varied levels of challenge for each student. For example, in the My Book section of WiggleWorks teachers can provide each student with a different writing suggestion using the recorded "teacher message" (see Figure 5.14). Ranging from highly structured to open-ended, tasks can require greater or lesser degrees of independent text generation.

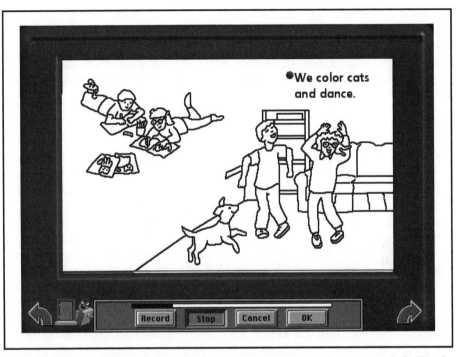

We color cats and dance.

Record Stop Cancel OK

Figure 5.14. WiggleWorks My Book with teacher message (being recorded). Teachers can record messages with individualized writing instructions for each student in WiggleWorks. *Note.* Screen shot from WiggleWorks Scholastic Beginning Literacy System. Copyright 1994 by Scholastic. Used with permission.

Examples of recorded teacher messages with different levels of structure include the following:

- Color the pictures and substitute your name for the word *we* on each page.

- Think of a new animal to color, put in the word, and draw a picture to go with it.

- Use your *My Words* list to place new words in the story.

- Use the *Record and Playback* button to record your ideas, then type the words to match. Click on the circle to hear your words read aloud, then compare them to your recording. Rewrite the words until they sound acceptable.

- Erase the words and picture, make a new story, and draw a new picture to go with it.

Many programs supporting multimedia composition are open ended, enabling teachers to establish varied levels of challenge by customizing the assignments according to students' skill levels and by encouraging students to use images and sounds in the completion of their work. Examples include HyperStudio (1994), Digital Chisel (1994–2000), and Imagination Express (1994).

Software That Offers Varied Supports

If setting the level of challenge correctly is one half of finding a student's zone of proximal development, the other half is providing the appropriate supports, or scaffolds. While the best scaffold is another person who can relate directly to the learner, computers can provide some wonderful and varied supports that extend a learner's reach. These include spell checkers, word prediction, voice recognition, wizards, prompts, help menus, and multimedia tools. Many of these have been addressed above in connection with their support of pattern recognition and strategy learning. Yet all are also critical for teaching to the ZPD and supporting engagement.

Spell checkers, for example, can enable students to produce more accurate documents and may at the same time help them develop spelling skills. Spell checkers compare the words in a word-processed document with words in a dictionary embedded in the word processor. They identify words that do not match the dictionary as misspelled words and offer suggestions for the correct spelling. After selecting a new spelling from the list, writers can substitute it for the original word with a keystroke. Spell checkers can be set up to check during writing or to analyze a completed or partially completed text on request. For students with learning disabilities, spell checkers may provide support, but may also bring some difficulties (MacArthur, Graham, Haynes, & DeLaPaz, 1996). They find both false negatives (e.g., proper names that are spelled correctly but are not in the dictionary) and false positives (words that are in the dictionary but are incorrectly spelled for the context in which they are placed, as often happens with homonyms). Further, because students with learning disabilities often produce spellings very far from correct, spell checkers may not "figure out" what a student was trying to spell, and therefore fail to generate the correct spelling. Spell checkers also tend to produce lists of esoteric words, which are difficult for students with learning disabilities to read or recognize. Because these students often have habitual misspelling patterns (i.e., spell by their own rules), they may not be able to recognize the correct spelling from a list of alternatives (see Figure 5.15).

Still, spell checkers have utility for students with learning disabilities. MacArthur et al. (1996) summarized an earlier study showing that students with learning disabilities corrected 36% of their spelling errors using a spell checker. Though this number appears discouragingly low, many of these stu-

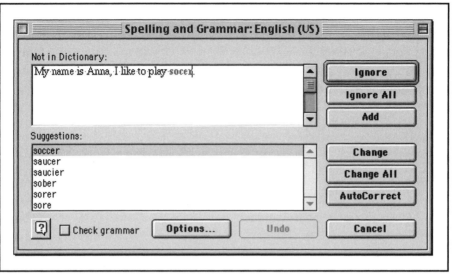

Figure 5.15. Microsoft Word spell check. Spell check requires students to choose the correct spelling from a list of possible words. *Note.* Screen shot from Microsoft Word. Copyright 1983–1998 by Microsoft Corp. All rights reserved. Used with permission.

dents typically fail to correct any of their own errors. Spell checkers that read the alternatives aloud can be enormously helpful for students with learning disabilities. Examples include Co:Writer (1993), SpellTools (for Macintosh), Planet.Speller (for Windows 1990), and Aurora for Windows (1997–1999). Particularly with text-to-speech, spell checkers support students in learning to self-evaluate their work and also to produce more accurate writing.

Voice recognition, mentioned in connection with strategy support, scaffolds text entry, and when combined with TTS feedback, can provide a highly supported environment for getting thoughts and ideas into textual form. Appropriate use of an array of supports can enable students to produce compositions independently and simultaneously increase awareness of the structures and procedures of different kinds of writing. These tools can be customized or used selectively for targeted goals, thus helping teachers individualize and keep each student engaged. Writer's Helper (1997) works with different word processors and provides support for all of the stages of writing via menus that generate prompts and elicit responses. Completed "notebooks" can then be exported to a word processor where Writer's Helper can support revision and editing (see Figure 5.16).

Multimedia itself can be used in a structured way to individualize supports and engage young writers. Students who have difficulty with text can generate a composition in images or sounds first, thereby building enthusiasm and

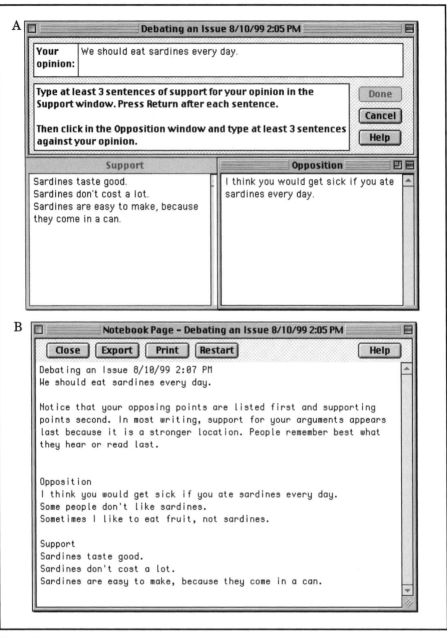

Figure 5.16. Writer's Helper in mid-composition (see A), and the finished product (see B). Writer's Helper can support the process of writing, helping students stay engaged in challenging tasks. *Note.* Adapted from Writer's Helper (Ver. 4.0 for Macintosh). Copyright 1989, 1996 by William Wresch. Published by Prentice Hall. Used with permission.

tapping into their creativity. Teachers, peers, and technology-based text-generating supports can then help them to compose in words (Leu, 1994, 1996; Meyer & Rose, 1998).

Software That Offers Timely and Relevant Feedback

Ongoing feedback is essential for engaging writers at all levels. Direct reactions from readers help students see their work as others do. Feedback helps students monitor their own effectiveness as communicators and evaluate their success in meeting their own goals or the aims of an assignment. Computers offer opportunities for both kinds of feedback in a timely way.

Text-to-speech (TTS), discussed for its value as a self-monitoring support, can also engage students' interest and motivation. Simply hearing the computer "read" back their work gives many students an emotional boost and encourages more editing and revising. Hollywood (1995), a program for creating digital animated "films," uses TTS to excellent advantage during the composing process. Students select characters and scenes, develop plots, write stage directions and dialogue, create a narrative sequence, and add music and sound. While composing, students can switch between edit and performance mode and watch and hear their films being enacted on the screen. In this way they can immediately evaluate the effect of their composition in terms of its dramatic outcome (see Figure 5.17). Hollywood is a highly engaging, creative tool which draws students into composing and promotes self-evaluation with immediate, powerful feedback.

The networked world of computers provides access to a very powerful source of feedback: responses from others (Leu & Leu, 1997). Taking the publishing stage of process writing to a new level, the posting of compositions on the Web brings an instant potential worldwide audience. Australian 6-year-old Alexander Balson, with help from his father, created a Web site, Alex's Scribbles: Koala Trouble, which has received almost 300,000 visits as of this writing. The site includes stories, drawings, music, e-mail exchanges, and links to Alex's favorite sites (see Figure 5.18).

Designing and posting a multimedia Web site is highly motivating for students with writing difficulties, even with limited outside response. During CAST's summer program, students with moderate to severe writing problems work enthusiastically for long hours creating their own personal Web sites on a variety of topics.

Technology That Sparks Personal Interest

In two studies of successful adults with dyslexia, Fink (1995, 1998) found in almost every case that her subjects had been avid readers in a subject of passionate personal interest as children and young adolescents, even though

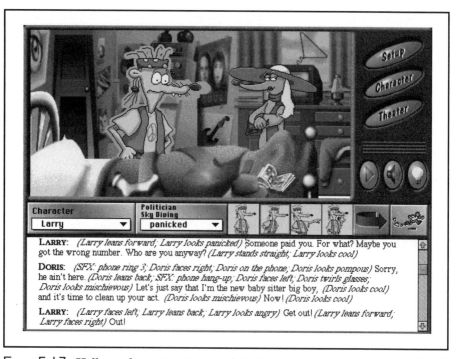

Figure 5.17. Hollywood uses text-to-speech technology engagingly to create digital animated "films." *Note.* Screen shot from Hollywood. Copyright 1995 by Theatrix Interactive. Used with permission.

they had not mastered the mechanics of reading. In the case of a significant minority of her subjects, difficulties with reading and writing mechanics persisted into adulthood; however, in many cases, these adults with dyslexia not only read extensively, but also wrote extensively in their professional lives.

The accessibility of hugely varied content is facilitated by CD-ROM libraries and the vast resources of the World Wide Web. Using digital media and networks, teachers can individualize subject matter for reading and writing to an extent not possible with print resources alone. As Fink's (1995, 1998) research suggests, passionate interest in a particular subject is a strong motivator. With on-line text sources such as On-Line Books Page (http://www.cs.cmu.edu/books.html), and Project Gutenberg (http://www.promo.net/pg/) or (http://www.gutenberg.net), it is now practical for teachers to individualize reading and writing subject matter content to a very great extent.

Critically important for success is careful selection and structuring of access to material. Simply "turning students loose" on the Internet and hop-

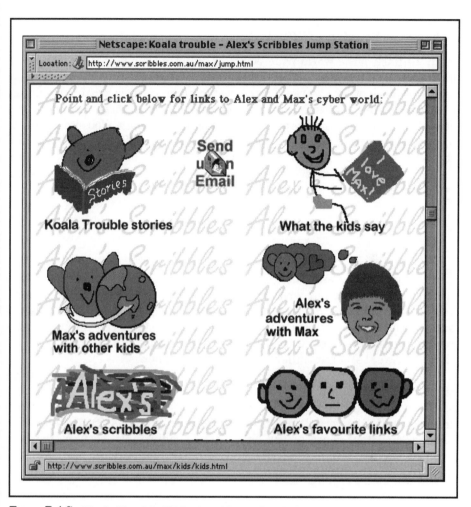

Figure 5.18. Koala Trouble Web site. Alexander Balson's illustrated stories have attracted worldwide attention. *Note.* Screen shot from Alex's Scribbles: Koala Trouble Web site. Available online: http://www.scribbles.com.au/max/jump.html. Copyright 1996–1999 by Alexander and Scott Balson. Used with permission.

ing they will find interesting and relevant material would not yield the desired results. A good way to structure access and help students stay focused is to create a home page with links to relevant material by subject area. Existing library and reference sites do just this and can be used as is or used as a model for teachers to create their own resource links (e.g., Internet Public Library at http://www.ipl.org/youth/).

Variable Learning Contexts

With the flash of the World Wide Web, it is sometimes easy to forget the power of simple e-mail, a highly motivating writing context. Students exchange e-mail with each other at a rapid rate, producing much more writing than they otherwise would. Web sites can also generate ongoing e-mail exchanges and stimulate writing. For example, at the Monster Exchange Web site, students draw wild monsters and then describe them in words. Correspondents read the descriptions and generate their own drawings from the text. Both motivating and fun, this exercise builds concise writing and careful reading skills (see Figure 5.19).

Conclusion

The concept of universal design for learning and the development of new technologies for teaching writing to students with learning deficits are both still in their infancy. Much more research is needed, both in the laboratory and in the classroom, before we will fully understand the complex inter-related mental processes involved in learning to write and the multiple ways that individual students differ in their skills and needs.

It is clear, however, that when teachers mindfully focus their efforts on the three essential elements of the brain's function in writing—recognition, strategy, and affect—they maximize their chances of reaching each student in a classroom of diverse learners. By combining different software tools, Web sites, and content sources, looking always for adjustable features, teachers can provide individualized learning opportunities for developing writers.

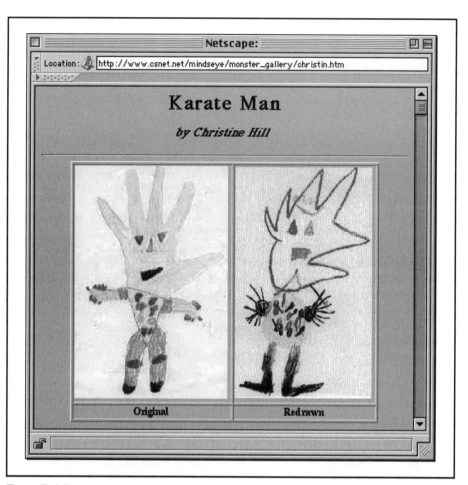

Figure 5.19. On the Monster Exchange Web site, children can draw wild creatures and then describe them in words for others to recreate from the description. *Note.* Screen shot from Monster Exchange Web site. Available online: http://www.csnet.net/mindseye/monster. Copyright by WinStar Communications. Used with permission. Browser window from Netscape Communicator. Copyright 1999 by Netscape Communications Corp. Used with permission.

References

Amazing Writing Machine [Computer software]. (1994). Novato, CA: Brøderbund.

Anderson-Inman, L., & Horney, M. (1996–1997). Computer-based concept mapping: Enhancing literacy with tools for visual thinking. *Journal of Adolescent & Adult Literacy, 40*(4), 302–306.

Anderson-Inman, L., Knox-Quinn, C., & Horney, M. (1996). Computer-based study strategies for students with learning disabilities: Individual differences associated with adoption level. *Journal of Learning Disabilities, 29*(5), 461–484.

Anderson-Inman, L., Redekopp, R., & Adams, V. (1992). Electronic studying: Using computer-based outlining programs as study tools. *Reading and Writing Quarterly: Overcoming Learning Difficulties, 8*(4), 337–358.

Anderson-Inman, L., & Zeitz, L. (1993, August/September). Computer-based concept mapping: Active studying for active learners. *The Computing Teacher*, pp. 6–11.

Anderson-Inman, L., & Zeitz, L. (1994, May). Beyond notecards: Synthesizing information with electronic study tools. *The Computing Teacher*, pp. 21–25.

Athey, I. (1976). Reading research in the affective domain. In H. Singer & R. Rudell (Eds.), *Theoretical models and processes of reading*. Newark, NJ: International Reading Association.

Aurora for Windows (Version 3.0) [Computer software]. (1997–1999). Burnaby, British Columbia, Canada: Aurora Systems.

Bahr, C. M., Nelson, N. W., & Van Meter, A. M. (1996). The effects of text-based and graphics-based software tools on planning and organizing of stories. *Journal of Learning Disabilities, 29*(4), 355–370.

Bailey's Book House [Computer software]. (1995). Redmond, WA: Edmark.

Bain, A. M. (1976). Written expression—The last skill acquired. *Bulletin of The Orton Society, 26*, 79–95.

Bardine, B. (1997). *Working with learning disabled writers: Some perspectives*. Bowling Green, OH: Kent State University.

Blakemore, S. J., Rees, G., & Frith, C. D. (1998). How do we predict the consequences of our actions? A functional imaging study. *Neuropsychologia, 36*(6), 521–529.

Burgess, P. W., & Shallice, T. (1996). Response suppression, initiation, and strategy use following frontal lobe lesions. *Neuropsychologia, 34*(4), 263–273.

Butkowsky, I. S., & Willows, M. (1980). Cognitive-motivational characteristics of children varying in reading ability: Evidence for learned helplessness in poor readers. *Journal of Educational Psychology, 72*, pp. 408–422.

Butler, D. L. (1995). Promoting strategic learning by postsecondary students with learning disabilities. *Journal of Learning Disabilities, 28*(3), 170–190.

CAST eReader [Computer software]. (1997). Peabody, MA: CAST.

Cermak, S. A. (1991). Somatodyspraxia. In A. G. Fisher, E. A. Murray, & A. C. Bundy (Eds.), *Sensory integration: Theory and practice* (pp. 137–168). Philadelphia: F. A. Davis.

Chapman, D. (1991). *Vision, instruction, and action*. Cambridge, MA: MIT Press.

Chapman, J. W., & Boersma, F. J. (1979). Academic self concept in elementary learning disabled children: A study with the Student's Perception of Ability Scale. *Psychology in the Schools, 16*, 201–206.

Cicci, R. (1980). Written language disorders. *Bulletin of The Orton Society, 30*, 240–251.

Cooper, R., & Shallice, T. (1997). *Modelling the selection of routine action: Exploring the criticality of parameter values*. Paper presented at the 19th Annual Conference of the Cognitive Science Society.

Co:Writer (Version 2.1.2) [Computer software]. (1993). Wauconda, IL: Don Johnston.

Csikszentmihályi, M. (1997). *Finding flow: The psychology of engagement with everyday life*. New York: Basic Books.

Cytowic, R. E. (1996). *The neurological side of neuropsychology*. Cambridge, MA: MIT Press.

Damasio, A. R. (1994). Descartes' error and the future of human life. *Scientific American, 271*(4), 144.

D'Arcangelo, M. (1998). The brains behind the brain. *Educational Leadership, 56*(3), 31–35.

Digital Chisel (Version 2.1.4) [Computer software] (1994–2000). Portland, OR: Pierian Spring Software.

Duffield, J. S., de Silva, R. N., & Grant, R. (1994). Pure alexia without agraphia: A classical cortical syndrome revisited. *Scottish Medical Journal, 39*(6), 178–179.

Elfgren, C. I., & Risberg, J. (1998). Lateralized frontal blood flow increases during frequency tasks: Influence of cognitive strategy. *Neuropsychologia, 36*(6), 505–512.

Ellis, E. S. (1998). Watering up the curriculum for adolescents with learning disabilities: Part 2. Goals of the affective dimension. *Remedial and Special Education, 19*(2), 91–105.

Englert, C. S., & Raphael, T. E. (1988). Constructing well-formed prose: Process, structure, and metacognitive knowledge. *Exceptional Children, 54*(6), 513–520.

Englert, C. S., Rozendal, M. S., & Mariage, M. (1994). Fostering the search for understanding: A teacher's strategies for leading cognitive development in 'zones of proximal development.' *Learning Disability Quarterly, 17*(3), 187–204.

Erdem, S., & Kansu, T. (1995). Alexia without either agraphia or hemianopia in temporal lobe lesion due to herpes simplex encephalitis. *Journal of Neuroophthalmology, 15*(2), 102–104.

Fink, R. P. (1995). Successful dyslexics: A constructivist study of passionate interest reading. *Journal of Adolescent & Adult Literacy, 39*(4), 268–280.

Fink, R. P. (1998). Literacy development in successful men and women with dyslexia. *Annals of Dyslexia, 48*, 311–346.

Ganschow, L. (1983). Analysis of written language of a language learning disabled (dyslexic) college student and instructional implications. *Annals of Dyslexia, 34*, 271–284.

Gershberg, F. B., & Shimamura, A. P. (1995). Impaired use of organizational strategies in free recall following frontal lobe damage. *Neuropsychologia, 13*(10), 1305–1333.

Goel, V., & Grafman, J. (1995). Are the frontal lobes implicated in "planning" functions? Interpreting data from the Tower of Hanoi. *Neuropsychologia, 33*(5), 623–642.

Goel, V., Grafman, J., Tajik, J., Gana, S., & Danto, D. (1997). A study of the performance of patients with frontal lobe lesions in a financial planning task. *Brain, 120*, 1805–1822.

Hallenbeck, M. J. (1995, April). *The cognitive strategy in writing: Welcome relief for adolescents with learning disabilities*. Paper presented at the Annual International Convention of the Council for Exceptional Children, Indianapolis, IN.

Heyman, W. B. (1990). The self-perception of a learning disability and its relationship to academic self-concept and self-esteem. *Journal of Learning Disabilities, 23*(8), 472–475.

Higgins, E. L., & Raskind, M. H. (1995). Compensatory effectiveness of speech recognition on the written composition performance of postsecondary students with learning disabilities. *Learning Disability Quarterly, 18*(2), 159–174.

Hollywood [Computer software]. (1995). Emeryville, CA: Theatrix Interactive.

Howard, P. J. (1994). *The owner's manual for the brain: Everyday applications from mind-brain research*. Austin, TX: Leornian Press.

Huntington, D. D., & Bender, W. N. (1993). Adolescents with learning disabilities at risk? Emotional well-being, depression, suicide. *Journal of Learning Disabilities, 26*(3), 159–166.

HyperCard [Computer software]. (1991). Cupertino, CA: Apple Computer.

HyperStudio [Computer software]. (1994). El Cajon, CA: Roger Wagner.

Imagination Express (Version Destination: Neighborhood) [Computer software]. (1994). Redmond, WA: Edmark.

Inspiration (Version 5.0) [Computer software]. (1997). Portland, OR: Inspiration Software.

IntelliTalk [Computer software]. (1993). Novato, CA: IntelliTools.

Jeannerod, M. (1997). *The cognitive neuroscience of action*. Cambridge, MA: Blackwell.

Jensen, E. (1998). How Julie's brain learns. *Educational Leadership, 56*(3), 41–45.

Johnson, D. H., & Myklebust, H. R. (1978). *Learning disabilities: Educational principles and practices*. New York: Grune & Stratton.

Karni, A., Meyer, G., Rey-Hipolito, C., Jezzard, P., Adams, M. M., Turner, R., & Ungerleider, L. G. (1998). The acquisition of skilled motor performance: Fast and slow experience-driven changes in primary motor cortex. *Proceedings of the National Academy of Sciences, USA, 95,* 861–868.

Koob, G. F., Cole, B. J., Swerdlow, N. R., & leMoal, M. (1990). *Stress, performance, and arousal: Focus on CRF* (Vol. Monograph No. 97-163176). La Jolla, CA: Research Institute of Scripps Clinic, Department of Neuropharmacology.

LeDoux, J. (1996). *The emotional brain: The mysterious underpinnings of emotional life*. New York: Simon & Schuster.

Leu, D. (1994, June). *Designing hypermedia to connect reading and writing through children's literature*. Paper presented at the National Education Computing Conference, Boston.

Leu, D. J. (1996). Exploring literacy within multimedia environments: Sarah's secret. *The Reading Teacher, 50*(2), 162–165.

Leu, D. J., & Leu, D. D. (1997). *Teaching with the Internet: Lessons from the classroom*. Norwood, MA: Christopher-Gordon.

Lewis, R. B., Graves, A. W., Ashton, T. M., & Kieley, C. L. (1998). Word processing tools for students with learning disabilities: A comparison of strategies to increase text entry speed. *Learning Disabilities Research & Practice, 13*(2), 95–108.

MacArthur, C. A. (1996). Using technology to enhance the writing processes of students with learning disabilities. *Journal of Learning Disabilities, 29*(4), 344–354.

MacArthur, C. A. (1998). Word processing with speech synthesis and word prediction: Effects on the dialogue journal writing of students with learning disabilities. *Learning Disability Quarterly, 21*(2), 151–166.

MacArthur, C. A., Graham, S., Haynes, J. B., & DeLaPaz, S. (1996). Spelling checkers and students with learning disabilities: Performance comparisons and impact on spelling. *Journal of Special Education, 30*(1), 35–57.

Malone, T. W. (1981). Toward a theory of intrinsically motivating instruction. *Cognitive Science, 4,* 333–369.

Malone, T. W. (1984). What makes computer games fun? Guidelines for designing educational computer programs. In D. Peterson (Ed.), *The intelligent schoolhouse*. Reston, VA: Reston.

Martin, K. F., & Manno, C. (1995). Use of a check-off system to improve middle school students' story compositions. *Journal of Learning Disabilities, 28*(3), 139–149.

Mavis Beacon Teaches Typing Version 10 Deluxe [Computer software]. (1999). Novato, CA: Brøderbund.

Meltzer, L. (1991). Problem-solving strategies and academic performance in learning-disabled students: Do subtypes exist? In L. V. Feagans, E. J. Short, & L. J. Meltzer (Eds.), *Subtypes of learning disabilities: Theoretical perspectives and research* (pp. 163–188). Hillsdale, NJ: Erlbaum.

Meyer, A. (1983a). *Competence, perceived competence, self-esteem and task persistence in learning-disabled children.* Unpublished doctoral dissertation, Harvard Graduate School of Education, Cambridge, MA.

Meyer, A. (1983b, July). Origins and prevention of emotional disturbances among learning disabled children. *Topics in Learning & Learning Disabilities*, pp. 59–70.

Meyer, A., Pisha, B., & Rose, D. (1991). Process and product in writing: Computer as enabler. In A. M. Bain, L. L. Bailet, & L. C. Moats (Eds.), *Written language disorders: Theory into practice.* Austin, TX: PRO-ED.

Meyer, A., & Rose, D. H. (1998). *Learning to read in the computer age* (Vol. 3). Cambridge, MA: Brookline Books.

Meyer, A., Rose, D., & Pisha, B. (1994). Out of print: Literacy in the electronic age. In N. J. Ellsworth, C. N. Hedley, & A. N. Baratta (Eds.), *Literacy: A redefinition* (pp. 55–59). Hillsdale, NJ: Erlbaum.

Microsoft Word 98 [Computer software]. (1998). Redmond, WA: Microsoft.

Morrison, G. M., & Cosden, M. A. (1997). Risk, resilience, and adjustment of individuals with learning disabilities. *Learning Disability Quarterly, 20*(1), 43–60.

My Words [Computer software]. (1993). Dimondale, MI: Hartley Courseware.

Naturally Speaking [Computer software]. (1997). Newton, MA: Dragon Systems.

Osherson, D., Perani, D., Cappa, S., Schnur, T., Grassi, F., & Fazio, F. (1998). Distinctive brain loci in deductive versus probablistic reasoning. *Neuropsychologia, 36*(4), 369–376.

*Out*SPOKEN (Version 1.7) [Computer software]. (1992). Berkeley, CA: Berkeley Systems.

Palincsar, A. S., & Klenk, L. (1992). Fostering literacy learning in supportive contexts. *Journal of Learning Disabilities, 25*(4), 211–229.

Petersen, S. E., van Mier, H., Fiez, J. A., & Raichle, M. E. (1998). The effects of practice on the functional anatomy of task performance. *Proceedings of the National Academy of Sciences, USA, 95*(3), 853–860.

Pisha, B. (1993). *Rates of development of keyboarding skills in elementary school aged children with and without identified learning disabilities.* Unpublished doctoral dissertation (University Microfilms #9326324), Harvard University Graduate School of Education, Cambridge, MA.

Planet.Speller [Computer software]. (1990). Atlanta, GA: The Planet Group.

Pompian, N. W., & Thum, C. P. (1988). Dyslexic/learning disabled students at Dartmouth College. *Annals of Dyslexia, 38*, 276–284.

Posner, M. I., & Raichle, M. E. (1994). *Images of mind.* New York: Scientific American Library.

Pullis, M. E. (1988). Affective and motivational aspects of learning disabilities. In D. K. Reid (Ed.), *Teaching the learning disabled: A cognitive developmental approach* (pp. 77–96). Boston: Allyn & Bacon.

Raviv, D., & Stone, A. C. (1991). Individual differences in the self-image of adolescents with learning disabilities: The roles of severity, time of diagnosis, and parental perceptions. *Journal of Learning Disabilities, 24*(10), 602–629.

Robin, N., & Holyoak, K. J. (1995). Relational complexity and the functions of the prefrontal cortex. In M. S. Gazzaniga (Ed.), *The cognitive neurosciences* (pp. 987–997). Cambridge, MA: MIT Press.

Roit, M. L., & McKenzie, R. G. (1985). Disorders of written communication: An instructional priority. *Journal of Learning Disabilities, 18*(5), 258–260.

Rourke, B. P., & Fisk, J. L. (1981). Socio-emotional disturbances of learning disabled children: The role of central processing deficits. *Bulletin of the Orton Society, 31,* 77–88.

Rubin, H., & Liberman, I. Y. (1983). Exploring the oral and written language errors made by children with learning disabilities. *Annals of Dyslexia, 33,* 111–120.

Schultz, W., Dayan, P., & Montague, P. R. (1997). A neural substrate of prediction and reward. *Science, 275,* 1593–1599.

SpellTools (Version 1.3.3) [Computer software]. (1995–2000). Wichita, KS: Newer Technology.

Stillwell, J. M., & Cermak, S. A. (1995). Perceptual functions of the hand. In A. Henderson & C. Pehoski (Eds.), *Hand function in the child: Foundations for remediation* (pp. 55–80). St. Louis, MO: Mosby.

Swanson, H. (1988). Toward a metatheory of learning disabilities. *Journal of Learning Disabilities, 21*(4), 196–209.

Sylvester, R. (1998). Art for the brain's sake. *Educational Leadership, 56*(3), 31–35.

Tomlinson, C. A., & Kalbfleisch, M. L. (1998). Teach me, teach my brain: A call for differentiated classrooms. *Educational Leadership, 56*(3), 52–55.

Type To Learn [Computer software]. (1992). Pleasantville, NY: Sunburst Communications.

ViaVoice [Computer software]. (1998). Armonk, NY: International Business Machines.

Vygotsky, L. (1962). *Thought and language.* Cambridge, MA: MIT Press.

Wallis, G., & Bülthoff, H. (1999). Learning to recognize objects. *Trends in Cognitive Sciences, 3*(1), 22–31.

Wetzel, K. (1996). Speech-recognizing computers: A written-communication tool for students with learning disabilities? *Journal of Learning Disabilities, 29*(4), 371–380.

White, J. L., Moffitt, T. E., & Silva, P. A. (1992). Neuropsychological and socio-emotional correlates of specific-arithmetic disability. *Archives of Clinical Neuropsychology, 7*(1), 1–16.

WiggleWorks Scholastic Beginning Literacy System [Computer software]. (1994). New York: Scholastic.

Wolfe, P., & Brandt, R. (1998). What do we know from brain research? *Educational Leadership, 56*(3), 8–13.

Wong, B. Y. L., Butler, D. L., Ficzere, S. A., & Kuperis, S. (1996). Teaching low achievers and students with learning disabilities to plan, write, and revise opinion essays. *Journal of Learning Disabilities, 29*(2), 197–212.

Write:OutLoud [Computer software]. (1994). Wauconda, IL: Don Johnston.

Writer's Helper (Version 4.0) [Computer software]. (1997). Upper Saddle River, NJ: Prentice Hall.

Writer's Solution: Writing Lab [Computer software]. (1997). Upper Saddle River, NJ: Prentice Hall.

Zipprich, M. A. (1995). Teaching web making as a guided planning tool to improve student narrative writing. *Remedial & Special Education, 16*(1), 3–15.

Ziviani, J. (1995). The development of graphomotor skills. In A. Henderson & C. Pehoski (Eds.), *Hand function in the child: Foundations for remediation* (pp. 184–196). St. Louis, MO: Mosby.

Curricular Strategies for Written Expression

<subsection>Barbara W. Gould</subsection>

W riting is a highly complex form of communication that permeates all aspects of the school curriculum; it is a cognitive act that requires formal instruction to develop. After taking a brief look at the kinds of problems students with learning disabilities encounter when they write, this chapter outlines a continuum of instructional approaches and suggests a variety of strategies that teachers can use to help these students.

Writing Problems of Students with Learning Disabilities

Students with learning disabilities can experience problems in almost any area of written expression. Although they may have good ideas, they often have difficulty using written language to convey them (D. Johnson & Myklebust, 1967; Myklebust, 1973; Poplin, Gray, Larsen, Banikowski, & Mehring, 1980) or to generate stories (Barenbaum, Newcomer, & Nodine, 1987). Because they may have difficulty understanding how others will perceive their writing (Bos & Filip, 1984), adapting to different audiences is often difficult for students with learning disabilities (Nodine, 1983). They often have trouble planning what to say, organizing how to say it, and monitoring how well they are doing (Englert & Raphael, 1988). Writers who have difficulty may be unable to retrieve words (German, 1979) or connect the different parts of their writing (Raphael, Kirschner, & Englert, 1988), and they are often preoccupied with mechanical details (Temple & Gillet, 1984). It is hard for them to edit their own work (Deshler, 1978). Students with learning disabilities compound these problems by using fewer types of words than other students (Morris & Crump, 1982) and writing less (Barenbaum et al., 1987; Myklebust, 1973), even when they have not exhausted their relevant knowledge. Unfortunately, by writing less, they write less well. (See Chapter 4 of this book for a more comprehensive discussion of written language disorders.)

Ways of Looking at Written Language

The past two decades have witnessed the emergence of important new ways of viewing written language, ways that offer alternatives for teaching students with learning disabilities. Drawing on Piaget and others, Britton (1972) suggested a natural sequence of development through three modes of functions and language. Expressive writing, which conveys the writer's thoughts and feelings, is the first to develop. This is the writing like speech, and it is from this base that the other two divergent forms develop. Transactional writing, issued to inform, explain, or persuade, is the next to develop. In poetic writing, the last to emerge, writing is a creative form, an end in itself. School writing has little to do with this sequence. Writing assignments in the early grades are mostly of a transactional and creative nature; least assigned are the expressive forms, which are the most natural for students (Whale & Robinson, 1978).

Combining Britton's ideas with an analysis of what people do when they write (Emig, 1971; Murray, 1980) has given rise to research on children's writing and an approach to teaching that directs attention to the process of writing (e.g., Britton, Burgess, Martin, McLeod, & Rosen, 1977; Calkins, 1983; Emig, 1971; Graves, 1983; Martin, D'Arcy, Newton, & Parker, 1976). This approach builds on communicative intent as the basis for writing. Students who have something to say and a reason for saying it are motivated to write, and they are motivated to learn to adapt their written forms to suit different audiences and circumstances. When students with learning disabilities have a reason to write, and when they do so not in response to teacher-driven exercise but to communicate with a receptive audience, their writing improves (Stires, 1983).

Curricular Choices: Isolated Skill Versus Holistic Approaches

Curricular choices extend across a broad spectrum, ranging from traditional, skill-centered, product approaches, which emphasize discrete outcomes and value writing only in terms of the final product, to newer, holistic, process-oriented approaches, which develop skills within the context of writing and value the learning that occurs during the process of writing (Rhodes & Dudley-Marling, 1988). Both are concerned with developing competence in writing, but they approach the teaching of it in different ways. Each approach emphasizes certain aspects of writing. Although the product approach provides for direct teaching of skills, it does not always ensure that students are able to transfer these skills to their own writing. The process approach, on the other hand, provides ample context for the application of skills, but does not adequately support students who have difficulty learning skills that have not been explicitly taught.

This continuum of learning approaches needs to be combined and integrated for the most effective instruction. Learning disabilities differ in degree and type from one student to the next. Students with mild handicaps may be able to learn, in part, through incidental approaches to skills development, whereas those with more severe deficits of attention, memory, motor, or language require direct, systematic skill instruction.

Isolated Skill Approaches

Based on the assumption that a skill is learned more easily in isolation before being merged and integrated with others, product-oriented curricula emphasize mastery of discrete skills, accentuating what F. Smith (1982) called the "secretarial skills" of written language: handwriting, spelling, and syntax. Traditionally, texts for teaching students with learning problems have followed this pattern (e.g., Hammill & Bartel, 1978; Mercer & Mercer, 1985; Wallace & Kauffman, 1986), giving only cursory attention to Smith's composition or authoring skills.

The desired integration does not always occur, however (Barenbaum, 1983; Sherwin, 1969). Emphasizing skills through repetitive writing tasks may hinder the learning process more than enhance it (Dyson, 1986; Poplin, 1984). Emphasis on skill mastery has given rise to the "red-pen" phenomenon, in which students' communicative intent is overlooked, and compositions and reports are often returned "bleeding from the margins having been marked profusely with red ink. "An overemphasis on correction may lead to writing styles characterized by safe, repetitive, and frequently unimaginative sentences . . . while coincidentally having a negative effect on student attitudes toward writing in general and toward creative production in particular" (Wallace, Cohen, & Polloway, 1987, p. 323).

Traditional, skill-oriented writing instruction measures student work against an ideal model that will always show the student to be deficient; in fact, the role of teachers in this approach is largely to indicate these deficiencies to their students. This model perpetuates the myth that good writers somehow magically produce a finished, flawless product, almost in a single step. For students with learning disabilities whose ideas, like those of all writers, are at first disorganized and jumbled, and who additionally lack either the skills or the confidence to put them together, the idea model may be overwhelming. Some of these students respond with fear and avoidance, writing as little as possible.

Holistic Approaches

Holistic curricula center on learning *through* the process of writing. Because students develop skills within the context of the writing, the sequence in which skills are taught develops, not in a preconceived plan, but in response to student needs. Writing instruction is structured, but the structure comes from the demands of the writing process and allows individuals to proceed at their own pace.

Going from an initial idea to a finished product is messy, rife with ambiguity and choices. The teacher's role is that of facilitator, guiding, encouraging, and teaching students as they work their way through the process. After helping students discover their ideas, teachers help them clarify and formulate these ideas, help them find solutions to their writing problems, and teach them the skills and strategies they need to organize their mess and to express their ideas coherently. Researchers and practitioners working with a general population of students have found that this approach increases both the quantity and quality of student writing while simultaneously building student confidence (Atwell, 1987; Calkins, 1986; Graves, 1983) and improving student attitudes toward writing (McHugh, 1986).

Despite evidence for the benefits of a process orientation, little research has been done involving students with learning disabilities. One study supporting the process approach for these students combines several orientations and recommends the structured teaching of skills within the context of a writing process environment (Gaskins, 1982). A study by Graham and Harris (1989) suggests that direct teaching of strategies for generating, framing, and planning text improves the writing of students with learning disabilities.

Components of Writing

Curricular strategies in this chapter are organized around four interacting components, or levels of writing, that make it possible to interpret and construct written language: background knowledge, semantics, syntax, and graphosymbolics. Based on a framework used to structure reading (May, 1986), these four components provide a convenient way of classifying writing strategies, and in so doing, they help connect and reinforce knowledge in both reading and writing. (A somewhat similar approach was taken by Rhodes & Dudley-Marling, 1988.)

Background Knowledge

Background knowledge is the accumulated knowledge and experience readers and writers possess. It provides schemata that readers activate as they read a passage; and it is the source of writers' material, shaping and defining what they can say about a topic. When writers' knowledge of a topic is meager, their ability to express ideas is limited; when they have topics that build on their knowledge, they can draw on their reservoir of information and experience to manipulate, organize, and clarify their ideas.

The desire to communicate information is at the heart of all language. When teachers capitalize on this desire and encourage students to share their knowledge with others, students not only begin with their expertise, but also with a reason to write. In the process, they learn about their subjects while developing writing skills. The semantic, syntactic, and graphophonic (graphosymbolic) systems of writing may all pose problems for students with learning disabilities. By drawing on the uniqueness of each student's background, teachers can make this one area a resource, an area of strength, a starting point.

Semantics

Both broad areas of semantics—text organization and vocabulary—can pose problems for writers with learning disabilities, who must be able to organize their thoughts coherently and retrieve the words that convey their ideas.

Syntax

Writers group words into phrases and sentences that follow predictable patterns. Even in a nonsense sentence, "The iggle oggled the uggle," the actor, action, and recipient are known, as are the patterns for changing the form of the sentence to a negative or a question, for example. The ability to use word forms correctly and to choose compatible forms is necessary for clarity. The ability to manipulate, expand, connect, and alter these patterns adds variety and interest to a writer's text.

Graphosymbolics

The most mechanical of the components requires production of graphemes and punctuation marks, which convey the message in a form that allows it to be retrieved and understood. Writers with learning disabilities often experience difficulty with spatial organization, handwriting, spelling, rules of capitalization, or punctuation. Word processors, spell check programs, and tape recorders can provide viable alternatives for some of these students.

Achieving success as a writer involves integrating the levels of language organization and processing into a cohesive whole. The sum of the whole is greater than the sum of the parts. The strategies in this chapter recognize both the desirability of learning skills in context and the need to isolate skills for instructional emphasis. Methods are grouped under the four main components of writing, beginning with the process-oriented, holistic strategies that emphasize students' background knowledge. Various methods for developing semantics and syntax in writing are then discussed. Lastly, issues related to writing mechanics, particularly as they affect the written composing process, are presented. Some teaching methods have been developed specifically for those with hearing losses and with learning disabilities. Other strategies and techniques that were originally developed to assist normally achieving students have been included because they have potential for helping students with learning disabilities as well. Since the needs of disabled learners vary widely, teachers are encouraged to combine and adapt the techniques to best fit their own students.

Stages of Writing

Observations of successful writers provide insight into the stages of writing and suggest that students need regular times to write, a sense of authorship and involvement, and a way to share their writing with others (Atwell, 1987; Calkins, 1983, 1986; Graves, 1983). As they write, authors go through several stages; prewriting (rehearsal), drafting (writing), and revision (rewriting), moving through the stages recursively (Emig, 1971; Flower & Hayes, 1984; Murray, 1980) before editing (proofreading), and sometimes also publishing (preparing for publication) their work. Each of these steps can be made explicit to students.

Prewriting (Rehearsal) Stage

The process of writing begins in the mind as writers first generate their thoughts and ideas, and then mentally plan what they will write. Drawing on their own experiences, interests, and knowledge, writers need to feel they have something worthwhile to say. As writers decide on their goal and think about their audience, they begin to connect their ideas (Murray, 1980) and tentatively organize their writing, mentally rehearsing what they are going to say and how they are going to say it. Students with learning problems can be shown how to increase their competence in selecting topics and planning their writing (Graves, 1983).

Students unaccustomed to choosing their own writing topics often have difficulty thinking of things to say. "Children who are fed topics . . . as a steady diet . . . rightfully panic when topics have to come from them" (Graves, 1983, p. 21). Students often overlook what they see as mundane and commonplace but nevertheless are "authorities on subjects they think are ordinary" (Murray, 1979, p. 16). When students' interests are identified and nurtured, students become increasingly willing to write.

Class discussions and conferences with the teacher or another student can help students identify topics. Students with learning disabilities often need extra help in identifying topics and may respond well to picture stimuli. Students who are taught to record topic ideas in their writing folders and to add new ideas as the occur, can compile a reservoir of suggestions for future use. Establishing a routine in which students spend the first minutes of each day writing in ungraded journals focuses attention on writing and encourages students to think of things to write about. These journal entries can often help students recall experiences or ideas suitable for expanded topics.

Teachers who know their students' backgrounds and interests can help them discover the value of what they know. Through discussion and gently probing questions, teachers can guide their students to discover and talk through topics, helping them identify and plan what they have to say. As students become more familiar with the process, they can interview each other; and then as students talk about their own topics, they can begin to rehearse what they will say (Calkins, 1986).

Through modeling both topic selection and initial planning, teachers can make these processes explicit for students. Thinking out loud and mulling over several ideas before settling on one idea provides a model of the process by which writers select topics. The process of verbally brainstorming what to say, identifying the intended audience, and making overt choices about what to include and what to exclude makes students aware of what writers do as they preplan their writing. Following the modeling with a group discussion in which students discuss their ideas for topics may be sufficient stimulation for some students. Others, like those with learning disabilities, may need more structure. For them, a review of the processes in the models can be used as the basis for identifying and teaching the specific steps involved. (Refer also to the section on developing written semantics for more structured organizational strategies.)

Drafting (Writing) Stage

The emphasis in this stage is on moving ideas from memory to paper, developing thoughts and constructing meaning, and gaining control over ideas, without worrying about form. Recursion is common in this stage as writers stop to think, plan, and rehearse what they will say next. Putting their ideas down on paper is often difficult for students with learning disabilities.

To ease this transition from thought to writing, teachers can encourage the verbal rehearsal begun in the previous stage and can free students from concerns about making mistakes. Special colored paper, stickers, or stamps that clearly identify the writing as unfinished at the outset can alleviate some concern about making mistakes. Oversized paper may make writing easier for some writers. Encouraging students to guess at spellings or to leave a blank space when they cannot think of a word fosters independence and helps them learn strategies that let them focus on thinking. Skipping spaces between lines leaves more room for later revision, making this next stage a little easier.

Daily writing in journals is especially important for students with learning disabilities who do not yet have a sense of flow when they write (Alley & Deshler, 1979). Initially, students write freely whatever comes to mind. When freed from the pressure of outside scrutiny, they can begin to feel successful about their writing, a feeling that teachers can encourage by writing personal responses sensitive to the content and intent of each student's work. By encouraging students to write in the expressive form that is most like speech (Britton, 1972), journals allow students to think about writing for different purposes and to learn from it in the same way they learn from speech (Martin et al., 1976). Later on, journal entries may become more focused as students respond to particular events or ideas. Teachers can again use modeling to let students observe the thought processes that accompany the transition from thought to paper, explicitly teaching the steps for those who need more structure.

Some students with learning disabilities may profit from dictating their own work, participating in the writing process unencumbered by the mechanics of inscription.

> [Taped talk] . . . retains all the advantages of talk whilst adding some of the advantages which traditionally have belonged to writing. Tape can be kept, it can be listened to any number of times, it can be transcribed, discussed, even redrafted and revised." (Martin et al., 1976, p. 50)

Language experience that builds on students' interests, ideas, and experiences (Allen, 1976; Stauffer, 1970) can serve as an introductory or transitional step for writers as well as for readers. After students identify a topic, discuss it, and plan what they want to say about it, they can dictate their ideas to a teacher or a peer recorder.

The steps following dictation depend on each student's level of competence. For students with more severe disabilities, someone can read the text back to them, eliciting the students' ideas for changes, revisions, and new drafts. Alternatively, the person can take notes for authors who prefer to as they make the changes themselves. Others may be able to process the dictated text, making their own revisions. In this way students continue to develop many writing skills despite handicaps in some areas.

Revision (Rewriting) Stage

Once ideas are down on paper, writers can look at what they have written in light of their audience and purpose. They can then begin to refine the meaning of what they have constructed, deciding what to change and what to keep. The decision to revise rests with the authors, and at first students do not revise their work at all. When they start to make corrections, they tend to concentrate on mechanical changes (Graves, 1979). It is not until they begin to think about their writing and to anticipate how a reader will respond that they begin to make changes in meaning. Teachers can facilitate the revision process by providing realistic audience feedback and by directly teaching skills that ease the process.

Because student writers know what they mean, they sometimes assume others understand as well. A group conference in which writers share their work enables them to see their writing from another's perspective. These revision conferences lend themselves well to small groups of peers, who listen as writers read their material out loud. The audience provides each writer with positive feedback, helping the writer discover what is good in the writing. Naive writers often do not know what is good or lack the confidence to trust their own judgment. By asking questions about the parts they have not understood, the audience can also help writers become aware of ambiguities and consider revisions to clarify their ideas.

Using brief, focused lessons to teach students revision shortcuts, such as crossing out unwanted parts and using carets, brackets, and arrows to rearrange and insert material, can make the process easier, reducing some of the students' reluctance to make changes. Even those who dread the mechanics of writing can learn to cut and paste. When students realize that working drafts do not have to be neat, they may be less fearful about writing and making changes.

Editing (Proofreading) Stage

Once writers are satisfied with the content of what they have said, they are ready to proofread and edit their work, making these final corrections on their working draft. Since changes in meaning have already been dealt with, the more mechanical skills are the primary focus of proofreading.

Initially, students identify and correct the errors they can, marking any areas where they think they need help. Some students may profit from the mnemonic device, COPS, an acronym for checking Capital letters, Overall appearance, Punctuation, and Spelling (Schumaker et al., 1981).

Since checklists are helpful guides in this process, students with special needs often benefit from individualized checklists tailor-made to reinforce the skills they know without feeling overwhelmed. High-priority skills are those essential to the writer's meaning or those that occur with considerable frequency (Graves, 1983). In general, when checklists begin with only a few items, students are more likely to pay attention to them. Gradually the number of items can be increased or upgraded. However, students with learning disabilities need to be taught how to use checklists, learning how to check sequentially and focus on just one item at a time.

As in the other stages, the goal is for students to steadily increase their skills, not necessarily to produce a flawless product. This approach that emphasizes developing mastery is more positive than one that measures students' work against a perfect standard. To emphasize their progress, students can make a chart of the skills they know, including spelling words and punctuation and capitalization rules (Bos & Vaughn, 1988).

When they have done as much as they can independently, students may ask a peer for help, confer with their teacher, or turn their paper in for review. Unfortunately, peers may become overly judgmental when they edit, and the time needed for editing conferences with the teacher may overshadow the other stages of writing (Calkins, 1986). This leaves the realistic option of handing work in to the teacher.

Teachers make additional corrections on the rough draft to help bridge the gap between accepted practice and the student's level of expertise. In some cases, teachers may indicate the location of an error, leaving the correction to the student; other times, the teacher provides the correction for the student; and in some instances, the teacher may choose to leave an error alone. Teacher editing requires sensitivity to each student's needs, an appreciation of the student's purpose for writing, and an understanding that when new skills are learned, they tend to be overgeneralized at first.

To help develop needed skills, directed lessons are frequently required. In addition, editing strategies can be taught either to the whole class or to small groups of students who are ready to use them. Learning to use proofreading marks can be an efficient and effective way for students to indicate the need for corrections on their paper and get a sense of control over their writing. The strategies taught can be very simple, limited to crosshatching to delete parts, circling or underlining to indicate words of uncertain spelling, boxes to indicate uncertain punctuation, arrows and brackets to move a section, and carets to mark insertions. Depending on the students' level of expertise, the traditional proofreading marks can be incorporated as the need arises, including the marks for deletion, capital and lowercase letters, paragraphs, and margins.

Publishing (Recopying) Stage

Once a work is edited, students may produce a polished version, recopying their work neatly or typing it in final form. This step is taken more for the sake of appearance, ease of reading, and pride of authorship, than for further learning; and it is *not* necessary for students to publish every piece they write. The motivation for students to publish their work is closely tied to their purpose for writing. If writers want someone to read what they have written, their work needs to be in readable form.

Edited work stays in a student's writing folder and can be retrieved for publication at a later time. Once several pieces have accumulated, writers may choose one piece to put in polished form. When students publish, the form they choose will depend on their audience. Sometimes writers illustrate their work or bind the pages of their writing together, covering them with a hard backing to form a book. A class newspaper provides another vehicle for publishing.

Guides to the Writing Process

Two programs, the Expository Writing Program (EWP) (Raphael et al., 1988) and Cognitive Strategy in Writing (CSIW) (Englert & Raphael, 1988; Englert, Raphael, Anderson, et al., 1988), use a series of think sheets to guide students through the writing process. CSIW, which is designed for children with special needs, incorporates teacher modeling and thinking aloud as well.

The think sheets focus students' thinking at each step of the process and, through a series of questions and prompts, actively engage them in planning. The prewriting planning sheet reminds students to consider their audience, their own knowledge, and ways to include and order their ideas. The organizing sheets vary according to the type of text structure. For example, the EWP compare/contrast sheet asks students to identify what they are comparing, to determine the dimensions of comparison, and then to list how the items are alike and different. The editing sheets help students analyze their work after they have used the prewriting and organizing sheets to write their rough draft. Students rate the content, clarity, and organization of their text, and in the EWP, they specify parts that need revision. A second editing sheet asks a peer to evaluate the text in a similar fashion. In EWP a final revision sheet is used for students to summarize the suggestions and indicate the changes they will make.

Applying Cognitive Strategy Instruction and Mnemonics to the Writing Process

Harris and Graham (1996) have found teaching students to use self-directed prompts with the writing process is effective in getting students to write more and to express themselves more effectively. Students are taught cognitive strategies for regulating their behavior along with specific strategies for writing. The development of these self-regulatory skills involves teaching students to set goals, to monitor progress, to assess and record results, to reinforce their behavior, and to use verbal self-directions to focus or refocus behavior (Harris & Graham, 1996, chap. 5).

By breaking the process of writing into small, manageable steps and using mnemonics, students can learn a variety of strategies for writing. Each strategy begins by developing background knowledge and discussing the goals of the strategy. It is then explicitly taught through detailed modeling of the writing strategy using those cognitive strategies that students can use for self-regulation. Students memorize the steps of the strategy along with any mnemonic prompt. Practice, at first carefully guided and structured, continues until students become more independent. Initially each strategy is taught in its most basic form. As students develop mastery, other components can be added one at a time, expanding the sophistication of both the strategy and the writing (Harris & Graham, 1996, p. 27).

One of the advantages of this approach is its flexibility and adaptability. Using cognitive strategies provides a framework that allows teachers to integrate structure and direct instruction with the writing process. Teachers can vary the amount of structure. They can focus on a single strategy, combine several strategies, or even tailor their own combinations of strategies to meet students' needs.

An example of the interaction between writing and the self-talk can be seen in the following five-step strategy designed to help students expand their use of vocabulary in their writing (p. 67).

- Think of a good story idea

- Write down good words for my story

- Write my story—use good words and make sure my story makes sense

- Read back over my story and ask myself—did I write a good story?

- Fix my story—can I use more good words?

By targeting specific kinds of words, like action or describing words, teachers can narrow the task and increase the structure.

Structured planning process helps students expand the quality of their writing. Setting specific, clear, attainable goals increases their chance of success. The mnemonic PLANS reminds students to Pick goals, List ways of meeting those goals, And make Notes, then Sequence the notes (Harris & Graham, 1996, p. 86).

TAP and Count is a strategy developed in Maryland that helps students grasp the basic components of writing. After identifying the writing Task, the Audience being addressed, and the Purpose for writing, students identify and number (Count) the main ideas or thoughts they want to include. Worksheets with numbered columns for each count help organize the process and provide room for notes. Depending on the complexity of the writing, each TAP may have one or more counts (Harris & Graham, 1996, pp. 124–129). A similar strategy used by many elementary teachers in Maryland is FAT P, a mnemonic prompting students to determine the Form, Audience, Topic, and Purpose. Part of the appeal of both strategies is their adaptability to a variety of genres and levels of writing complexity.

Another basic writing strategy is Think, Plan, and Write and Say More (Graham & Harris, 1989; Harris & Graham, 1996, p. 75). In step one, students consider why they are writing and who their audience will be. During planning, they identify what they want to say. "The third step [Write and Say More] is a reminder to the student to use the plans already devised and to continue the process of planning while writing" (Harris and Graham, 1996, p. 75). Taught initially for a single genre, students can later be shown how to generalize this strategy. Harris and Graham (1996) recommend using this strategy in conjunction with TREE and SPACE.

TREE can help students write a persuasive essay. It reminds them to (1) include a Topic sentence stating what they believe; (2) list the Reasons why they believe it; (3) Examine their reasons to be sure they are persuasive; and (4) End with a concluding sentence (Harris & Graham, 1996, pp. 76–79). Once students have mastered TREE, they can be introduced to STOP and DARE to expand the sophistication of their arguments. STOP reminds students to Suspend judgment and list pros and cons for both sides of a position, Take a side and select the best arguments to use, Organize the ideas and number the arguments in the order of use, and finally Plan more as they write (Harris & Graham, 1996, p. 82). DARE uses cue cards to prompt students to Develop a topic sentence, Add supporting ideas, Reject arguments for the other side, and End with a conclusion (pp. 82–83).

SPACE is a story-writing strategy that uses basic elements of story grammar. It includes Setting, physical and temporal, and identification of the main character; the main character's Purpose; the ensuing Action; the Conclusion; and the Emotions felt by the character (Harris & Graham, 1996, p. 76). Each component can be targeted and taught in detail to make the task more manageable. A slightly longer story mnemonic (p. 49) involves seven components: WWW What=2 How=2. This mnemonic reminds students to tell Who the main character is, When and Where the story takes place, What the main character does or wants to do, What happens, How the story ends, and finally How the main character feels. One way to introduce these strategies is by first teaching students to interpret and write about a picture using these mnemonics.

A modification of a strategy similar to K-W-L (described later in this chapter) uses webbing for writing reports instead of the traditional three columns (Harris & Graham, 1996, pp. 96–97). Using a web, children record what they already know about the topic and use question marks to indicate unknown or missing information. After gathering more information and making appropriate revisions, they use the web to start writing. As they write, they continue to plan what they are going to write, checking the web periodically to ensure they are sticking to their plan.

SCAN is one of several strategies that help students revise their written work. SCAN is appropriate for a persuasive opinion essay, but it can easily be adapted to other genres. First, students read their work. They find the sentence that tells what they believe, then check to be sure it is clear. Next, they add two more reasons why they believe that position. Then they SCAN the article sentence by sentence, checking each one to be sure it makes Sense, that it is Connected to what the writer wants to say, to Add more to what has already been said, and to Note any errors (Harris & Graham 1996, pp. 101–107).

Harris and Graham (1996) described Scardemelia and Bereiter's C-D-O strategy, which uses color-coded choice cards to help students revise their work during a Compare stage. Students evaluate a portion of their writing by choosing from among five blue cards with options ranging from "This doesn't sound right" to "This is good." They then move to a second pile of option cards to Diagnose the appropriate action, such as "Say more" or "Leave this the Same." The final step, Operate, translates diagnosis into writing (Harris & Graham, 1996, pp. 113–118). The complexity of this strategy can be controlled by varying the number of choice cards and, therefore, the number of options available.

A peer revision strategy allows pairs of students to help each other revise and proofread their papers. Students begin by reading their own papers orally to their partners, who listen and read along. The listeners tell what the paper is about and what they liked best. Students exchange papers and make notes on their partner's paper, using question marks to indicate lack of clarity and writing three suggestions for details that might be added. Students discuss their recommendations with each other before going back and making their own revisions (Harris & Graham, 1996, pp. 108–110). PODC is a peer revision device for secondary students. It reminds them to check to ensure that the basic Parts—beginning, middle, and end—are included, that the Order is logical, that Detail is added where more is needed or could be added, and that their writing is Clear (Harris & Graham, 1996, p. 113).

Another peer strategy, SCPS, guides pairs to proofread their work. Students first check their own papers and correct errors. They then exchange papers with their partner. Each partner checks Sentences for completeness, Capital letters at the beginning of sentences and proper nouns, and Punctuation at the end of the sentence. Questionable Spelling is circled for later checking. Partners discuss their findings with each other, before making their own corrections (Harris & Graham, 1986, pp. 108–110).

Of special value for students with learning problems is the combination of writing strategies with self-coaching techniques that help them define the problem, focus their attention, plan strategies, evaluate their work, cope with frustration, and provide reinforcement to themselves (Harris & Graham, 1996, p.139). Mnemonics are used in many of these strategies to help self-regulation. Other devices include cue cards to reduce the load on memory or colored choice cards to reduce the number of options. Charts, frames, webs, and other graphic organizers help focus attention on specific tasks. Checklists and worksheets can be combined with any of the strategies to provide additional structure and organization. Used together in a methodical, step-by-step progression, the combination of cognitive self-regulation with strategies for writing provides a powerful strategy for helping with written language difficulties. However, the writing strategies are not limited to that population. These strategies can help many children organize components of the writing process and, through specific step-by-step instruction, turn an abstract writing task into a much more manageable one.

Generating and Developing Writing Topics

Reading response logs represent a useful method to encourage writing, one that uses writing to stimulate thinking about reading. Not only is reading a resource that provides background information and concepts for writers, but also the two processes reading and writing interact and reinforce each other (Shanahan, 1988). As writers read and revise their writing, they begin to see themselves as authors and appreciate what authors do. As they critique their own writing and that of their peers, they learn to ask questions and critique the writing of others. As they learn to organize their writing and express themselves, they become aware of the rhetorical strategies of other authors.

These logs, either structured or unstructured, work equally well with content or fictional material and can be used at almost any grade level (Atwell, 1987; Calkins, 1986). Like other journals, they are neither edited nor revised, encouraging instead thinking and expression of ideas. If the log is unstructured, students, after reading, simply spend a few minutes entering their questions, thoughts, and feelings about the reading and providing a running commentary on their reactions. Regular and frequent entries not only stimulate thinking about the material but also help writers to become more fluent in their writing. Entries may be shared with a peer or with a group in class discussion, or they may be responded to privately in conversational comments written by the teacher.

Structured logs have a similar format, but the writing period is more controlled and may be better suited to students with learning disabilities who require greater structure. A specific writing period ranging from 3 to 15 minutes is set aside after reading for students to write in their journals. Teachers may design questions or prompts that focus on some aspect of the selection or help direct students' thinking in a specific way (Calkins, 1986).

For example, before beginning *Charlotte's Web* by E. B. White, students might respond to "What do you know about a spider?" or "If you were the author, how would you introduce a spider? Where would it be? What would it be doing?"

Prompts during the reading may emphasize significant aspects of the reading and may help students connect what they have already read with the reading still to come.

Questions at the end of a selection can elicit a general reaction to the story, invite a consideration of alternatives, or probe some aspect of the reading by posing prompts such as, "What would you tell a friend about this book?" or "Pretend you had written this story and you had it take place in a different location. Where would you put it?"

Entries may also be written in response to material read orally by the teacher (Atwell, 1987; Simpson, 1986) or to movies shown in class. These variations may have appeal for students with learning disabilities whose reading skills are limited.

Teacher-Selected Topics

Although research indicates that when students select their own topics the quality of their writing improves, students with learning disabilities may require more structure in this area. Some teachers prefer assigning topics around a common theme. One approach is for students to choose their own subtopics from a broader category selected by the teacher. An assignment on animals, for example, might spawn individual selections from seals to snakes. Projective topics, such as writing about a "most embarrassing event" or "the scariest event," may encourage students to write about their own experiences. Modifying a language experience approach, by having students write individually about a shared experience that has first been developed and discussed in a group, provides a more structured way of developing a common topic.

Developing Written Semantics

Semantic strategies are divided into two broad categories; organizational strategies and vocabulary. Both are areas that often pose problems for students with learning disabilities. Teachers may need to spend more time with these students in the prewriting stage, helping them develop their ideas and teaching them specific strategies to use as they plan and draft their work.

Organizational Strategies

Students with learning disabilities often have difficulty formulating their ideas and grouping and ordering these ideas for writing. This is compounded by the fact that the way ideas are organized varies from one text form to another, from one purpose to another, and from one audience to another.

Students with learning disabilities need additional structure to help them organize their ideas in a coherent manner. Many of the strategies in this section provide a visual framework for planning. Others are schema-based approaches that teach students how to deal with different text structures, an area that shows promise for helping students with learning disabilities in both reading and writing (Englert & Raphael, 1988; Englert, Raphael, Fear, & Anderson, 1988; Englert & Thomas, 1987; Rhodes & Dudley-Marling, 1988). A few more general strategies are also included.

The organizational strategies discussed in this section are divided into two groups: those primarily for narrative and story text, and those for content, descriptive, and expository material. However, the distinction between forms is not always clear, and Calkins (1986) suggested that authors often shift from one form to another.

Strategies for Narrative and Story Text

Narrative text is the most naturally occurring of the text structures and, in its simplest form, has a chronological order that young children can use in retelling their experiences (Calkins, 1986; Rhodes & Dudley-Marling, 1988). Writing stories becomes more complex as characters, settings, goals, problems, solutions, and outcomes are incorporated into the telling. The techniques that follow include suggestions for ordering ideas and for summarizing and creating story structures.

Sequence Strategies. Putting a series of pictures or cut-apart comics in chronological order may help students who have difficulty sequencing, but the writing that follows is likely to be artificial. Strategies that help students sequence their own ideas, such as time lines (Giordano, 1984) and flow charts, might have more impact. A time line indicating first, second, third, and so on, can be done on a large scale, adding physical distance to the time intervals, with events or steps written on index cards and placed on the time line. A flow chart, such as the one shown in Figure 6.1, or a chart with the prompts, first, second, third, and so forth, provide alternative outlines that students can refer to as they write.

Sequencing directions is a more difficult skill because of the need to see things from another's point of view. Additional feedback, such as that provided by peer conferencing, may be beneficial.

Modeling Story Elements. Teachers can use modeling both to make students aware of the different elements of story structure and to help them understand the malleability of these elements. Displaying a draft of their own story on an overhead projector, highlighting one aspect of it (character, setting, beginning), then thinking out loud about ways to vary that part, establish a model that students can apply to their own writing.

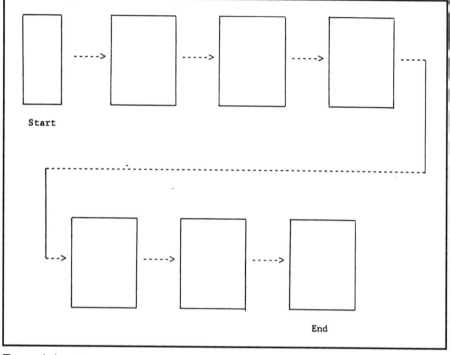

Figure 6.1. Flow chart for sequencing.

Story Outlines and Story Maps. Story outlines, chartlike structures that provide prompts for the different aspects of the story, are most valuable in helping students write summaries of existing stories, but they can also be used to help them plan their own stories. These prompts, in the form of questions or corresponding story elements (*who*—character; *when* and *where*—setting; *why*—goal), vary in length and complexity. The prompts can be expanded (first, second, etc.), and a second column can be added for listing details. Story maps are simple story outlines arranged in a more visual format as shown in Figure 6.2.

Story Frames. Story frames, or paragraphs with spaces for inserting words, phrases, or sentences, can help students to write summaries of stories they have read, to plan their writing, or to develop particular subsections (Nichols, 1980). The following sample frame was developed by Wood (1984, p. 497):

▶ **A story takes place _____. _____ is a character in the story who _____. A problem occurs when _____. After that, _____. Next, _____. The problem is solved when _____. The story ends _____.**

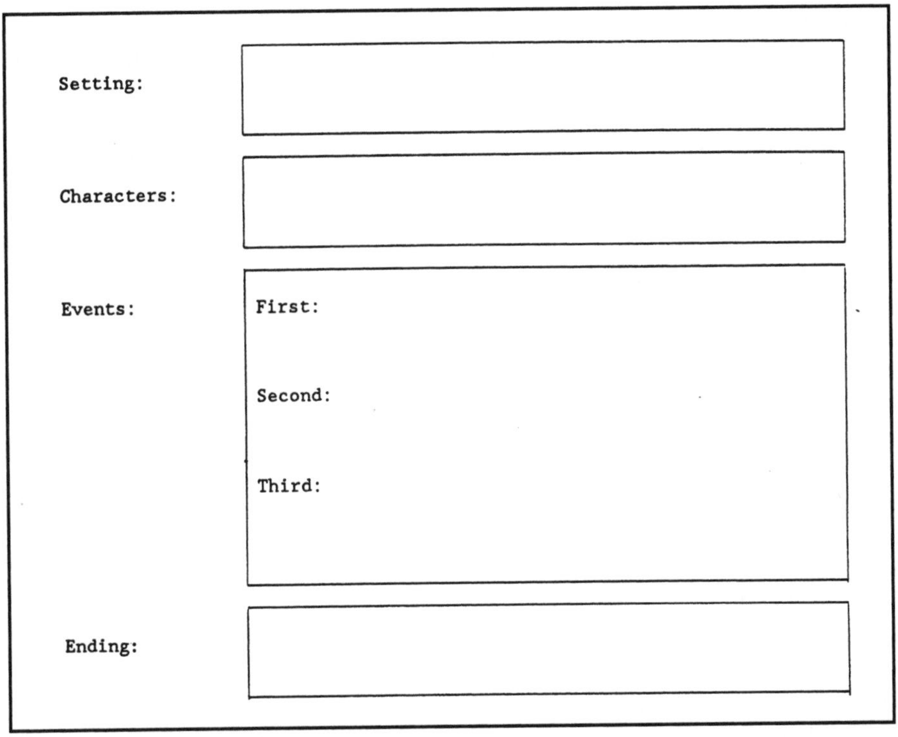

Figure 6.2. Story map. *Note.* Adapted from *Guaranteed To Work: Practices Which Promote Reading, Writing, and Thinking,* by Baltimore County Public Schools, 1988, Towson, MD: Author.

Probable Passages. Probable passages (Wood, 1984) is a combination of story outlines and story frames that integrates writing with reading comprehension. Teachers select key terms and phrases from a story to be read and present them to students along with copies of an outline of story elements (setting, characters, problem, problem solution, ending) and a story frame with spaces that correspond to the order of the items in the outline. Students first discuss the terms and phrases, then list them under the appropriate headings. Selecting one or more entries from each column of the outline or from their own background, they tentatively fill in the blanks of the story frame, working to construct a plausible story. After reevaluating their overall story logic and rearranging words and ideas to read smoothly, they can read the original passage and revise their own versions accordingly. Although probable passages are written initially with teacher guidance, after practice they can be constructed by small groups working together (Wood, 1984).

Detail Maps. Maps, similar to the semantic maps described later for vocabulary, can be used to help students develop specific parts of their story (character, setting, plot). A character map might put the character at the hub of a circle, with radiating spokes listing different traits; in a setting map, half the spokes might specify details of location, and the other half, details of time.

Macro-Cloze. In a macro-cloze exercise (Whaley, 1981), students are provided with copies of a passage in which one component (setting, beginning, reaction) is omitted and replaced with blank lines. After discussion, students either singly or in pairs construct a substitute for the omitted material. In a variation, students are divided into groups with each group given the same passage but each with a different section missing. When all groups are finished, the new sections are put together to create an original passage.

Strategies for Descriptive and Expository Text

Writing descriptive and expository texts in content areas requires research and organizational skills. Outlining and mapping strategies provide structures for gathering information, organizing it logically, and guiding the writing; other strategies ease the transition between outline and written draft.

Outlines and Charts. A box chart, which uses a spatial format to categorize main ideas and details, is one of the simplest strategies for writers. Designed for broad topics, box charts also allow students to select individual subtopics. Through discussion, students decide on significant questions, informational categories, or main ideas that pertain to the broad topic. With a sheet of paper divided into four to six equal boxes, one idea is put at the top of each box. Students complete each section by listing relevant information about their individual topics, using outside sources to add to or confirm their information. An assignment on mammals, for example, might use such categories as appearance (What does the animal look like?), food, habitat, enemies, young, and habits, which would provide the structure for subtopics from bats to whales. Each box becomes a separate paragraph in the text; if further structure is needed, the number of details and even the kind of details to include can be specified.

A more traditional outline form, which could serve as a transition for students ready to move beyond the box chart, lists the categories or questions on a sheet of paper, leaving room for details after each category (Hennings & Grant, 1981). Alternatively, a slightly more advanced data chart in the form of a grid of boxes can be used to introduce the concept of a research report. The categories or questions are used as column headings, with the left-hand column reserved for the names of two or three different sources, including oneself. The bottom row of boxes summarizes the findings in each category and becomes the referral source for the actual writing (Rhodes & Dudley-Marling, 1988).

As students become more independent, index cards can provide a flexible way to organize main ideas (Kucer, 1986). Students jot down major ideas associated with their topic, record them, one idea per card, and order them in a tentative outline, discarding some and adding others as needed. Sharing their cards with a peer who orders them independently may suggest alternative sequences as well as providing an awareness that outlines are subjective and tentative. The cards provide the basis for the development of each section of the paper. In the writing of independent reports, this approach needs to be coupled with reading and note-taking, although for students who need more support, it could be done as a classroom language experience activity.

Graphic Organizers. Graphic outlines, expository maps, and semantic webs are all graphic ways to connect and organize the ideas and information gained from reading (Horowitz, 1985b; L. L. Johnson, 1989; P. L. Smith & Tompkins, 1988; Wixon & Peters, 1985). Related to the semantic maps discussed earlier, these graphic organizers group major concepts into categories indicating their relationship to each other and provide a visual framework that students can use to write summaries or reports. Configurations vary, reflecting the structure of the text. L. L. Johnson (1989) recommended stars to represent conceptual relationships, trees to represent hierarchical ones, charts to compare similar concepts, chains to indicate sequence, and sketches to visualize descriptions; but others, including sunbursts, are possible.

K-W-L Plus. K-W-L is a charting strategy that actively involves readers with expository text (Ogle, 1986); K-W-L Plus extends this to writing (Carr & Ogle, 1987). The basic K-W-L technique has four components, three of which are indicated by the letters in the acronym. In the first step, students brainstorm and list in the first of three columns what they already Know, or think they know, about the topic (K). With teacher guidance, they think of pertinent categories of information and note them in a separate area at the bottom of the form. The second column consists of what they Want to find out (W), such as questions based on personal interest, ambiguities from column one, and categories for which there is inadequate information. At this point, students read to discover the answers to their questions and add information, noting in column three what they have Learned (L). In K-W-L Plus, the information in the third column becomes the basis for writing, the plus.

Text Frames. Text frames that reflect the basic structure of the text can help students make the transition between the organizational outlines and written expression. A sample descriptive frame might begin with a classification sentence followed by details:

▶ **A _____ is a mammal that looks _____. It has _____ and _____ and is _____.**

A comparison and contrast frame might incorporate cue words:

▶ **___1___ and ___2___ are both _____. They have _____ and _____, but ___1___ is _____ while ___2___ is _____. Although ___1___ _____, ___2___ _____.**

Frames for these and other structures can be developed through class discussion or provided by the teacher. In using this technique with students who have learning problems, the potential for confusion exists; therefore, it is recommended that teachers initially use the frames in conjunction with charts that first outline the relevant categories. This approach separates the task into its components and allows students to focus on one thing at a time.

Vocabulary Usage Strategies

The vocabulary available to writers is determined by three factors: the writers' familiarity with words, the depth of their conceptual understanding of those words, and their ability to retrieve words as needed. The vocabulary of students with learning disabilities may be limited; they frequently overuse general, nondescriptive words like *thing, goes,* and *does.* Even when these students know a more specific word, they may fail to recall it or may recall it inaccurately, substituting an associated word that conveys a different meaning. The concepts that underlie particular words may be incomplete or inaccurate. Students with these types of difficulties need strategies that broaden their vocabulary and provide access to more specific vocabulary that is appropriate to their meaning. They need help finding and retrieving the words they already know, and they need to know how to recognize and deal with these deficits in ways that minimize the impact on their writing.

Included in the strategies that follow are cue words that emphasize the relationship between transition words and the structure of the text, word lists and cloze activities that emphasize word awareness and retrieval, semantic feature analysis and semantic maps that emphasize conceptual understanding, and the use of dictionaries and thesauri as general references. Additional techniques for vocabulary development can be found in D. D. Johnson and Pearson (1984).

Cue Words

Explicit instruction may be necessary for students to understand the association between cue words and different forms of text structure and to learn to use these words to connect ideas and signal transitions. Horowitz (1985a) suggests *first, second, then*, and *next* to indicate chronological order; *first, in addition*, and *furthermore* for listing; *however, nevertheless,* and *on the other hand* for compare–contrast; *the cause, the effect, because, as a result, therefore*, and *consequently* for cause–effect; *the problem, the solution, the question*, and *the answer* for problem solving.

Word Lists

Word lists expand awareness of word choices and help with word retrieval problems, providing a measure of security for students faced with a blank sheet of paper as well as poor spelling skills. Lists can be developed through group discussion and displayed on charts or can be recorded individually, over time, in journals or on index cards. In some instances, such lists can even be provided by the teacher. As a general rule, developing vocabulary within the context of students' experiences eases and enhances the learning process (May, 1986).

Thematic lists developed around a particular topic provide an immediate reference for students to use in their writing. Categorical lists encourage more varied vocabulary by suggesting synonyms or alternatives for overused words or providing groups of action or descriptive words.

Hierarchical lists can help students see the relationships between words. Listing related words in order from specific to general or vice versa helps to clarify the relationships between superordinate and subordinate classes, an area of difficulty for some students with learning disabilities (Englert & Raphael, 1988). Placing the vocabulary words within a triangular shape with the most general word at the base adds visual impact and can be extended to sentences as well (Klein, 1985). In another form of hierarchical list, students rank related words, such as *weary, tired*, and *exhausted* or *squabble, quarrel*, and *feud*, according to their degree of severity, intensity, size, or some other attribute, thereby increasing the awareness of nuances (D. D. Johnson & Pearson, 1984).

Word lists can be used to create crossword puzzles for reinforcement. Computer programs like Crossword Magic (1985) arrange the words, reduce the complexity of puzzle design, and allow students to concentrate on designing clues for their entries.

Fill-ins

Blank spaces in the context of writing serve as either a strategy for writing or an exercise for expanding vocabulary. Teaching students to leave a space when a word does not come to mind is a drafting strategy that allows writers to continue their thoughts without interruption and return to the problems later. To expand vocabulary, teachers can cover up words from students' written work, and in small groups, encourage exploration of different possibilities. An alternative strategy substitutes antonyms instead of synonyms for key words, producing a version diametrically opposed to the original; advertisements or similar material are especially well suited to this type of exercise.

Semantic Feature Analysis

Analysis of the semantic features of words helps students compare similar words and clarify concepts in content areas (D. D. Johnson & Pearson, 1984), providing writers with greater precision in choosing specific vocabulary. Several words that share a common class (*soccer, basketball, baseball, lacrosse*) or are similar in meaning (*field, park, lawn, meadow*) are placed in a column on the left; columns on the right are headed by a general feature or characteristic that describes one or more of the words. The intersection of words and features forms a grid, which is then filled in with + symbols when words have an attribute and − symbols when they do not, providing a visual chart of similarities and differences. An extension of this idea, which goes beyond vocabulary development, uses this format to compare characters or events as a prewriting exercise.

Semantic Maps

Semantic maps provide a graphic way of exploring the relationships among words by categorizing them and connecting them to one another (Heimlich & Pittleman, 1986; D. D. Johnson & Pearson, 1984). In their most basic form, a central word is selected for mapping and written on an overhead or chalkboard. As students brainstorm for related words, the teacher records them and groups them in categories around the stimulus, visually creating spokes radiating from a hub. Students identify the categories exemplified by each spoke and discuss the relationships within and between the categories. Because they expand and structure thinking, maps can be used as a prewriting activity and as an aid to students who tend to focus on limited aspects of a concept.

Dictionaries and Thesauri

The dictionary and the thesaurus offer resources for writers who have difficulty moving beyond overworked terms or need help understanding nuances between words. Although they may be helpful in prompting synonyms for students with mild retrieval problems, the definitions are often too abstract to help students with more severe disabilities. In addition, learning to use these resources requires specific instruction and guidance. Having a range of elementary, high school, and collegiate dictionaries often proves useful because students can find a reference at their own comfort level. A personalized dictionary can also be helpful.

Developing Syntax Skills

Written grammar, putting words together to form written phrases and sentences, builds on students' oral syntactic development. Many students with learning disabilities experience difficulty acquiring the rules for forming sentences (D. Johnson & Myklebust, 1967). Problems in perception, memory, sequencing, processing, or concept formation may interfere with their ability to learn the rules that govern the acquisition of morphemes or with their ability to generate and use complex sentences.

In the early stages of speech, most children combine words, using nouns and verbs appropriately (Wiig & Semel, 1984), and by the time they enter school, they are familiar with basic sentence patterns (Loban, 1976). Children who experience delays or deviations in this sequence may need oral language intervention to develop a conceptual base that can then be reinforced and expanded through written language. (Refer to Wiig & Semel, 1984, for intervention strategies.)

Because "children [normally] . . . learn about language by using it" (DeHaven, 1983, p. 67), formal, rule-based grammar instruction that is isolated from the language that students use is not as effective in helping them improve their writing (Sherwin, 1969; Temple & Gillet, 1984) as instruction that develops these skills within the context of the students' own language. Such formal grammar instruction may even be detrimental if it displaces more appropriate writing instruction (Braddock, Lloyd-Jones, & Schoer, 1963).

This is not to say that students with learning disabilities do not need direct instruction in the area of syntax. Often direct instruction is the most effective means for identifying and teaching specific skills to those students. However, when the content of this instruction reflects the student's own language, and rules are taught within that context, there is greater promise for long-term learning (Barenbaum, 1983; Wiig & Semel, 1984).

The most common syntax errors are incorrect substitutions, additions, and omissions (Anderson, 1982), although one study found that many of the omissions resulted from oversight rather than lack of knowledge concerning the appropriate construction (Goodman, Casciato, & Price, 1987). Teachers need to provide strategies to help students deal with these errors. One way to help them identify and correct these errors is for teachers to identify the problems first, one type at a time, providing a written model of the correct form. Using the model as a guide, students then look for and correct other examples of that error (Rhodes & Dudley-Marling, 1988, pp. 159–160).

Words and Phrases

The instructional strategies in this section are designed to increase students' awareness of morphological forms and expand their knowledge of variations of these forms by focusing on a few at a time. In general, these strategies are recommended as teacher-led group activities.

Classification

Emphasis on particular kinds of words highlights their form and use. Word games are one approach that can be used. In one game, students construct sentences that repeat and exaggerate a form, then add an unexpected or contradictory ending (Temple & Gillet, 1984, pp. 236–237), for example, "The bird sailed, swooped, swayed, and soared, but never stopped."

Structured poetry that specifies word types can help students develop fluency with syntactic forms. A variation of a five-line poem, the cinquain, has 11 words specified as follows: one noun (line 1), two adjectives describing the noun (line 2), three *-ing* verbs describing the noun (line 3), a four-word descriptive phrase (line 4), and a noun related to the initial one (line 5).

Fill-ins and Substitutions

Filling in and substituting words or phrases is another way to highlight specific grammatical forms. Using examples from students' work provides additional reinforcement.

Cloze. A paragraph with cloze-type exercises can elicit words or phrases that highlight a particular function. The sentences "Bob _____ the ball" or "Bob threw the _____" prompt verbs and nouns; "Bob threw the ball _____ (where, how, when, or why)" or "The baseball player _____" prompt adverbial and verb phrases. Students who have difficulty generating these forms can learn by having to choose between two or three correct examples. Students ready for more challenge can have more blanks to complete in each paragraph, or complete blanks that call for a variety of word forms, or both.

Mad Libs. In a variation on the commercially available Mad Libs, the teacher provides a brief story, eliminating crucial words or phrases, and then numbers the missing words, indicating their form (e.g., prepositional phrase indicating location). With no knowledge of the original story, students decide on an appropriate type of word or phrase for each number. Inserting them in the blanks can provide an entertaining story.

Substitutions. While substituting words or phrases for existing ones is slightly more challenging than filling in blanks, it introduces a skill students need to correct their own work. At the easiest level, students suggest alternatives for a word or phrase. In the sentence, "Mary swam in the water," students can suggest alternatives for any one of three parts: *Mary, swam,* or *in the water*.

To help students apply substitution strategies to their own work, teachers can use a copy of students' work with different words, or types of words or phrases, covered with tape. Students then consider different possibilities for the deletions as in the cloze activity above (Giordano, 1984, p. 54; Rhodes & Dudley-Marling, 1988, p. 231).

Constructing Sentences

In order to construct basic sentences, students need to be able to recognize sentences, to put words in the appropriate order, and to insert words in sentences to yield more information. Strategies for enhancing each skill are discussed in turn.

Sentence Recognition

Strategies for increasing sentence recognition include using established sentence patterns, combining partial sentences, and distinguishing between sentences and not-yet sentences.

Patterns. For younger children, repeated word patterns in stories can serve as a model (Cox, 1988, p. 214). Predictable texts like Bill Martin's *Brown Bear, Brown Bear*, "Brown bear, brown bear, what do you see? I see a red bird looking at me," provide patterns that children can copy, yet can vary to create their own story. Add-on stories or song texts that use repeated patterns to add a new section, like Peppe's "The House That Jack Built" or Bonne and Mill's "I know An Old Lady" (who swallowed a fly . . .), provide a second type of model that teachers can use with students to add verses or to write parallel text.

Partial Sentences. Using teacher models, students can brainstorm and list separately noun phrases (*the little old lady*) and verb phrases (*jumped into the stream*), which they can combine to make either realistic or silly sentences (DeHaven, 1983, p. 233). As students gain more competence, they can generate their own complementary phrases when provided with a stimulus phrase.

Another approach for students who need more structure is to provide almost-completed sentences lacking only one or two words. Word by word, the number of prompts are gradually diminished, so that students are providing more of the sentence (Mercer & Mercer, 1985, p. 443).

Not-yet Sentences. Samples of phrases and sentences from students' work can be used in discussions to identify sentences and not-yet sentences and to elicit suggestions for turning the latter into sentences.

Sentence Expansion

Students can build sentences of increasing length and complexity by ordering and expanding a basic kernel sentence one part at a time. Beginning with a minimal noun–verb construction, they add words or phrases that fill specific form classes.

Sentence Order. Working individually or in pairs, students can build sentences from sets of index cards that have different classes of words or phrases written on them (Hennings & Grant, 1981, p. 173). This exercise can also be used to illustrate the fact that phrases can sometimes, but not always, occupy more than one spot in a sentence without changing the meaning. The noun phrases cannot be transposed in *"The little girl* opened *the heavy door,"* but in "The cars honk loudly *in the city,"* the location of the prepositional phrase is more flexible.

Several structured programs use visual prompts to develop specific types of expansions, building on the predictability of word order. The commercially available *Fokes Sentence Builder* (Fokes, 1976), designed for oral language, can be adapted for written language as well. Pictures are classified in color-coded boxes representing the following prompts: who, what, is doing, which, where, whose, how, and when. Students build sentences by arranging the pictures in the appropriate order. Montessori's (1973) writing program uses a carefully sequenced series of grammar boxes that group words of similar function together, coding them with symbols of varying colors, shapes, and sizes (e.g., nouns, articles, and adjectives are represented by triangles of three different colors and sizes). Sentence frames use the symbols in conjunction with question prompts to elicit specific word forms, and the student then copies the ensuing sentence. In the *Teaching Written Expression* program (Phelps-Terasaki & Phelps, 1980; Phelps-Terasaki, Phelps-Gunn, & Stetson, 1983), students write words and phrases in appropriate columns in response to questions from the teacher about a target sentence. For example, the teacher might ask, "Who is eating an apple?" "What is he doing?" and "What is he eating?" to elicit the target sentence "He is eating an apple."

Framing Your Thoughts (Greene & Enfield, 1993) is another written language program specifically designed for students with learning disabilities. This program teaches children to recognize a "barebone sentence." Children are taught to expand sentences and also to analyze them systematically by producing shape-coded sentence diagrams. This program moves slowly with a great deal of structured practice.

Descriptive Inserts. Words or phrases that serve as adjectives or determiners (articles, possessives, numbers) can be inserted to expand noun phrases, and those serving as adverbs can be inserted to expand verb phrases. Expanding each part separately, beginning with noun phrases that are easier, helps focus attention on the components; later they can be combined. For example, in the kernel sentence "Birds flew," *birds* and *flew* could be expanded to "The hungry birds in the tree" and "flew quickly to the food on the ground." When combined they yield, "The hungry birds in the tree flew quickly to the food on the ground." Students can create these expansions individually or as a game in a small group.

Teachers can lift sentences in need of expansion from students' work and, using carets to indicate target areas, generate suggestions in class discussion. To preserve the writer's integrity, each student has the final say in choosing which, if any, version to insert in the final work (Rhodes & Dudley-Marling, 1988).

Insert-a-Word Poems. A novel approach, which uses two-word kernel sentences to create brief, free-form poems, lends itself well to a group effort (Hennings & Grant, 1981, p. 177). Students begin by brainstorming and listing word pairs that follow the lead of a model provided by the teacher (e.g., *rabbits hop; children flop; toads plop*). Several such couplets can be put together and left as is, or they can be expanded by inserting a descriptive word (*fuzzy rabbits hop; tired children flop; jumpy toads plop;* or *rabbits nimbly hop; children wearily flop; toads clumsily plop*).

Combining Sentences

In order to write sentences that have variety and complexity, writers must be able to do more than simply expand sentences. Authors use a variety of techniques for joining, embedding, and rearranging phrases and sentences, and instruction in these techniques may help students who have difficulty in writing complex sentences to become more skilled (Faigley, 1980; Nutter & Safran, 1983, 1984; O'Hare, 1973).

Although prepared materials are available that provide sequenced instruction (Strong, 1986), actually lifting sentences from students' work to experiment with different combinations helps students determine which option is best and why, including the option not to combine at all (Rhodes & Dudley-Marling, 1988, pp. 231–232). Sentences with compound parts and those in which a single word is embedded are generally easier to produce than those that involve embedding of phrases and clauses. Characteristically, the writings of students with learning disabilities lack these complex embedded forms.

One way to approach combining is to begin with a stimulus sentence, preferably from students' writing, and have students generate similar sentences, changing one or more parts. Students then underline the overlapping parts and combine the sentences, deleting the repetition and making final adjustments. For example, the stimulus sentence (S), "Sally rides her bike to the store," might generate the following new sentences: (1) "Mary rides her bike to the store," (2) "Sally walks to the store," and (3) "Sally walks to the movies." Combining S and 1 entails joining two noun phrases with *and,* changing *her* to *their* and *bike* to *bikes* ("Sally and Mary ride *their* bikes to the store"). Because S and 2 are contradictory, the conjunctions *either, or,* or *but* are the most likely options for combining them; after deleting the redundancy, no further changes are necessary ("Sally *either* rides her bike *or* walks to the store"). The only overlap between S and 3 is the subject, and the verb phrases can be combined with either *and* or *but* ("Sally rides her bike to the store but walks to the movies").

A game reported by Hennings and Grant (1981, p. 183) begins with a list of verbs generated by the students. Working in pairs, the students write two sentences for one of the verbs. They then combine the sentences, deleting the redundant verb, and start again with another verb, trying to see how many combined sentences can be completed within a specified time.

Sentence Embedding

Embedding provides an efficient way for authors to relate thoughts within a sentence. Embedding, which is inserting a word, phrase, or clause from one sentence into another, involves multiple steps. Writers arrange remaining sentence fragments, decide where to place the embedded section in the new sentence, select or construct the means for inserting it (word, phrase, clause), and then make any necessary final adjustments.

Single words and phrases that can be moved intact with no change in wording are often easier than those that require the writer to rearrange, add, or change words. Clauses can function as adjectives ("The boy who ate the melon . . ."), nouns ("Jim knew what he wanted"), or adverbs ("When Sally saw the bike . . ."), depending on the word that introduces the clause and the relationship expressed. When children insert noun or adverbial (subordinate) clauses in oral language, they tend to put them at the end of sentences, although they may also insert subordinate clauses in such a way that the sentence order matches the chronological order of events ("After he fell, Bob went to the doctor") (Wiig & Semel, 1984, p. 472).

Whenever possible, samples from students' own writing can be used to teach embedding. Lifting suitable sentences from students' work, and brainstorming possibilities for combining them, develops an awareness of some of the ways in which phrases can be embedded. Reading the alternatives out loud may help determine which one to use. Underlining the section of a sentence to be embedded or indicating where to put it in the new sentence, and even providing the first word of a clause, reduces the complexity of the task and provides additional structure for those who need it.

In an exercise that isolates embedding from contextual writing, a teacher provides two lists. The first list consists of basic sentences; the second list contains noun and subordinate clauses. Students try to see how many sentences they can make by matching them (Hennings & Grant, 1981, p. 185).

Converting Sentences

Techniques for converting sentences from the declarative form to other forms (negative, question, passive, ellipsis) are more commonly found in oral language development than in written language. However, one highly structured approach, CATS, incorporates instruction in transformations as part of its instructional sequence.

Developed by Giordano (1982), CATS, an acronym for Copy, Alter, Transfer, Supply, is a four-step technique designed for writers with learning disabilities. A statement made by the student is recorded by the teacher, then copied verbatim by the student. ("I like candy.") The student alters one word of the sentence, and rewrites it. ("You like candy.") In response to teacher direction, the student transforms the sentence, changing its form or converting the tense of the verb, and writes the new sentence. ("I don't like candy." or "Do you like candy?") In the last step, the teacher writes a question, then the student supplies a written response. ("I like M&M's.") If necessary, the sentences written at each stage may be dictated orally by the student, then recorded and read by the teacher before actually being copied by the student.

Developing Graphosymbolic Skills

Developing the ability to use graphic symbols can be extremely challenging for some students with learning disabilities. Of the skills in the graphosymbolic area—handwriting, spelling, spatial organization, punctuation, and capitalization—the two most fundamental, handwriting and spelling, can pose the greatest problems. Because these areas are so complex, they require specialized teaching techniques, which are discussed fully in separate chapters. (See Chapters 1 and 2 of this book for a discussion of spelling and Chapter 3 for a discussion of handwriting.)

Punctuation and capitalization can be taught within the context of students' writing. There is increasing evidence that developing some of these mechanical skills within the context of the students' own writing provides for greater transfer of these skills. Strategies which teach these skills within the larger context of written expression may encourage students to write more. When students need skills to help them communicate a message in which they have a vested interest, this need creates a climate that motivates the learning. A class of third-graders who learned punctuation through the context of frequent writing understood twice as many punctuation marks (eight) as their counterparts who had been taught skills in isolation; not only that, but because they understood the need for the different forms of punctuation, they also enjoyed using them (Calkins, 1983, p. 35).

Lessons can teach one particular rule or review and emphasize several skills. Samples reproduced from class writing can lead to discussions of particular punctuation marks or rules governing the use of capital letters. Young children can be given cards with different punctuation marks on them, which they hold up or insert while a passage is being read orally or written on the board (Mercer & Mercer, 1985). Teachers can use their voice in conjunction with overhead transparencies to reinforce the impact of specific punctuation marks (Atwell, 1987). Students can classify capitalized words according to the reasons for their use (Mercer & Mercer, 1985). A review exercise in which all punctuation marks, capital letters, or both are removed from a passage can serve as the stimulus for students working in pairs or small groups.

When attention is focused on the mechanical aspects in the process of expressing ideas through written language, this focus may be to the detriment of the ideas. Poor writers are often preoccupied with mechanical skills too early in the writing process, effectively stifling their writing expression (Temple & Gillet, 1984, pp. 295–296). Delaying the emphasis on these skills until later allows students to focus first on their ideas and then give their attention to mastering some of the mechanical skills they need. Within this context, directed lessons that isolate and teach one specific skill at a time have the advantage of immediate and meaningful application to the students' own work, thereby increasing the likelihood of understanding, retention, and transfer.

Summary

Students with learning disabilities have difficulty attending simultaneously to multiple demands, yet writing demands multiple skills. To reduce the resulting conflict, making the process manageable for these students requires lessons that teach specific skills and an approach to writing that allows students to focus on one thing at a time.

To improve their writing, students need to write regularly and frequently. Since they write more when they have something they want to say, approaches that begin with students' knowledge and experiences and that teach writing as a process have been emphasized. Techniques for helping students learn the skills for generating and organizing their ideas, drafting and revising them, then editing and publishing them, have been included to provide a structure that allows students to focus on one aspect of the writing process at a time. Where possible, techniques that allow skills to be taught within the context of the students' writing have been emphasized.

Although there is not yet a large body of research showing the benefits of this approach for students with learning disabilities, there is much in the literature that makes it seem very promising for them.

References

Allen, R. V. (1976). *Language experiences in communication*. Boston: Houghton Mifflin.

Alley, G. R., & Deshler, D. D. (1979). *Teaching the learning disabled adolescent*. Denver, CO: Love.

Anderson, P. L. (1982). A preliminary study of syntax in the written expression of learning disabled children. *Journal of Learning Disabilities, 15*(6), 359–362.

Atwell, N. (1987). *In the middle: Writing, reading, and learning with adolescents*. Portsmouth, NH: Boynton/Cook.

Baltimore County Public Schools. (1988). *Guaranteed to work: Practices which promote reading, writing, and thinking*. Towson, MD: Baltimore County Public Schools.

Barenbaum, E. M. (1983). Writing in the special class. *Topics in Learning & Learning Disabilities, 3*(3), 12–20.

Barenbaum, E., Newcomer, P., & Nodine, B. (1987). Children's ability to write stories as a function of variation in task, age, and developmental level. *Learning Disabilities Quarterly, 10,* 175–188.

Bos, C. S., & Filip, D. (1984). Comprehension monitoring in learning disabled and average students. *Journal of Learning Disabilities, 17,* 229–233.

Bos, C. S., & Vaughn, S. (1988). *Strategies for teaching students with learning and behavior problems*. Boston: Allyn & Bacon.

Braddock, R., Lloyd-Jones, R., & Schoer, L. (1963). *Research in written composition*. Urbana, IL: National Council of Teachers of English.

Britton, J. (1972). Writing to learn and learning to write. In G. M. Pradl (Ed.), *Prospect and retrospect: Selected essays of James Britton* (pp. 94–111). Montclair, NJ: Boynton/Cook.

Britton, J., Burgess, T., Martin, N., McLeod, A., & Rosen, H. (1977). *The development of writing abilities*. Urbana, IL: National Council of Teachers of English.

Calkins, L. M. (1983). *Lessons from a child*. Portsmouth, NH: Heinemann.

Calkins, L. M. (1986). *The art of teaching writing*. Portsmouth, NH: Heinemann.

Carr, E., & Ogle, D. (1987). K-W-L plus: A strategy for comprehension and summarization. *Journal of Reading, 30*(7), 627–631.

Cox, C. (1988). *Teaching language arts*. Needham Heights, MA: Allyn & Bacon.

Crossword Magic [Computer software]. (1985). Northbrook, IL: Mindscape.

DeHaven, E. P. (1983). *Teaching and learning the language arts* (2nd ed.). Austin, TX: PRO-ED.

Deshler, D. D. (1978). Psychoeducational aspects of learning disabled adolescents. In L. Mann, L. Goodman, & J. L. Wiederholt (Eds.), *Teaching the learning-disabled adolescent* (pp. 48–74). Boston: Houghton Mifflin.

Dyson, A. H. (1986). Staying free to dance with children. *English Education, 18*(3), 135–146.

Emig, J. A. (1971). *The composing processes of twelfth graders* (Research Rep. No. 13). Urbana, IL: National Council of Teachers of English.

Englert, C. S., & Raphael, T. (1988). Constructing well-formed prose: Process, structure, and metacognitive knowledge. *Exceptional Children, 54,* 513–520.

Englert, C. S., Raphael, T. E., Anderson, L. M., Anthony, H., Fear, K., & Gregg, S. (1988). A case for writing intervention: Strategies for writing informational text. *Learning Disabilities Focus, 3*(2), 98–113.

Englert, C. S., Raphael, T. E., Fear, K., & Anderson, H. (1988). Students' metacognitive knowledge about how to write information texts. *Learning Disability Quarterly, 11,* 18–46.

Englert, C. S., & Thomas, C. C. (1987). Sensitivity to text structure in reading and writing: A comparison of learning disabled and non-learning disabled students. *Learning Disability Quarterly, 10,* 93–105.

Faigley, L. L. (1980). Names in search of a concept: Maturity, fluency, complexity and growth in written syntax. *College Composition and Communication, 31*(3), 291–300.

Flower, L. S., & Hayes, J. R. (1984). Problem-solving strategies and the writing process. In R. G. Graves (Ed.), *Rhetoric and composition: A sourcebook for teachers and writers* (pp. 269–282). Montclair, NJ: Boynton/Cook. (Reprinted from *College English, 39,* pp. 449–461, 1977)

Fokes, J. (1976). *Fokes sentence builder.* New York: Teaching Resources.

Gaskins, I. W. (1982). A writing program for poor readers and writers and the rest of the class, too. *Language Arts, 59*(8), 854–861.

German, D. (1979). Word-finding skills in children with learning disabilities. *Journal of Learning Disabilities, 12,* 176–181.

Giordano, G. (1982). CATS-exercises: Teaching disabled writers to communicate. *Academic Therapy, 18,* 233–237.

Giordano, G. (1984). *Teaching writing to learning disabled students.* Rockville, MD: Aspen.

Goodman, L., Casciato, D., & Price, M. (1987). LD students' writing: Analyzing errors. *Academic Therapy, 22*(5), 453–461.

Graham, S., & Harris, K. (1989). Improving learning disabled students' skills at composing essays: Self-instructional strategy training. *Exceptional Children, 56*(3), 201–214.

Graves, D. H. (1979). Research update: What children show us about revision. *Language Arts, 56*(3), 312–319.

Graves, D. H. (1983). *Writing: Teachers and children at work.* Exeter, NH: Heinemann.

Greene, V. E., & Enfield, M. L. (1993). *Framing your thoughts.* Bloomington, MN: Language Circle Enterprises.

Hammill, D. D., & Bartel, N. R. (1978). *Teaching children with learning and behavior problems* (2nd ed.). Boston: Allyn & Bacon.

Harris, K. R., & Graham, S. (1996). *Making the writing process work: Strategies for composition and self-regulation.* Cambridge, MA: Brookline Books.

Heimlich, J. E., & Pittleman, S. (1986). *Semantic mapping: Classroom applications,* Newark, DE: International Reading Association.

Hennings, D. G., & Grant, B. M. (1981). *Written expression in the language arts: Ideas and skills* (2nd ed.). New York: Teachers College Press.

Horowitz, R. (1985a). Text patterns: Part 1. *Journal of Reading, 28*(5), 448–454.

Horowitz, R. (1985b). Text patterns: Part 2. *Journal of Reading, 28*(6), 542–543.

Johnson, D., & Myklebust, H. R. (1967). *Learning disabilities: Educational principles and practices.* New York: Grune & Stratton.

Johnson, D. D., & Pearson, P. D. (1984). *Teaching reading vocabulary* (2nd ed.). New York: Holt, Rinehart & Winston.

Johnson, L. L. (1989). Learning across the curriculum with creative graphing. *Journal of Reading, 32*(6), 509–519.

Klein, M. L. (1985). *The development of writing in children: Pre-K through grade 8.* Englewood Cliffs, NJ: Prentice-Hall.

Kucer, S. B. (1986). Helping writers get the "big picture." *Journal of Reading, 30*(1), 18–24.

Loban, W. (1976). *Language development, kindergarten through grade twelve.* Urbana, IL: National Council of Teachers of English.

Martin, N., D'Arcy, P., Newton, B., & Parker, R. (1976). *Writing and learning across the curriculum.* London: Ward Lock Educational for The Schools Council.

May, F. B. (1986). *Reading as communication: An interactive approach* (2nd ed.). Columbus, OH: Merrill.

McHugh, B. (1986). Study examines effect of process approach. *Highway One, 9*(2), 80–86.

Mercer, C. D., & Mercer, A. R. (1985). *Teaching students with learning problems* (2nd ed.). Columbus, OH: Merrill.

Montessori, M. (1973). *The Montessori elementary material.* New York: Schocken Books. (Orginally published as *The advanced Montessori method,* Vol. 2, 1917)

Morris, N. T., & Crump, W. D. (1982). Syntactic and vocabulary development in the written language of learning disabled and non-learning disabled students at four age levels. *Learning Disability Quarterly, 5*(2), 163–172.

Murray, D. M. (1979). The listening eye: Reflection on the writing conference. *College English, 41*(1), 13–18.

Murray, D. M. (1980). Writing as process: How writing finds its own meaning. In T. R. Donovan & B. W. McClelland (Eds.), *Eight approaches to teaching composition* (pp. 3–20). Urbana, IL: National Council of Teachers of English.

Myklebust, H. R. (1973). *Development and disorders of written language: Studies of normal and exceptional children* (Vol. 2). New York: Grune & Stratton.

Nichols, J. N. (1980). Using paragraph frames to help remedial high school students with written assignments. *Journal of Reading, 24*(3), 228–231.

Nodine, B. F. (1983). Foreword: Process not product. *Topics in Learning & Learning Disabilities, 3*(3), ix–xii.

Nutter, N., & Safran, I. J. (1983). *Sentence combining and the learning disabled child.* (ERIC Document Reproduction Service No. 252–94).

Nutter, N., & Safran, I. J. (1984). Improving writing with sentence combining exercises. *Academic Therapy, 19,* 449–455.

Ogle, D. (1986). K-W-L: A teaching model that develops active reading of expository text. *The Reading Teacher, 39*(6), 564–570.

O'Hare, F. (1973). *Sentence combining: Improving student writing without formal grammar instruction* (Research Rep. No. 15). Urbana, IL: National Council of Teachers of English.

Phelps-Terasaki, D., & Phelps, T. (1980). *Teaching written expression: The Phelps sentence guide program.* Novato, CA: Academic Therapy.

Phelps-Terasaki, D., Phelps-Gunn, T., & Stetson, E. G. (1983). *Remedation and instruction in language, reading, and writing.* Austin, TX: PRO-ED.

Poplin, M. (1984). Toward a holistic view of persons with learning disabilities. *Learning Disability Quarterly, 7,* 130–134.

Poplin, M., Gray, R., Larsen, S., Banikowski, A., & Mehring, T. (1980). A comparison of components of written expression abilities in learning disabled and non-learning disabled children at three grade levels. *Learning Disability Quarterly, 3,* 46–53.

Raphael, T. E., Kirschner, B. W., & Englert, C. S. (1988). Expository writing programs: Making connections between reading and writing. *The Reading Teacher, 41*(8), 790–795.

Rhodes, L. L., & Dudley-Marling, C. (1988). *Readers and writers with a difference: A holistic approach to teaching learning disabled and remedial students*. Portsmouth, NH: Heinemann.

Schumaker, J. B., Deshler, D. D., Nolan, S., Clark, F. L., Alley, G. R., & Warner, M. M. (1981). *Error monitoring: A learning strategy for improving academic performance of LD adolescents* (Research Rep. No. 32). Lawrence: University of Kansas Institute for Research in Learning Disabilities.

Shanahan, T. (1988). The reading–writing relationship: Seven instructional principles. *The Reading Teacher, 41*(7), 636–647.

Sherwin, J. S. (1969). *Four problems in teaching English: A critique of research*. Scranton, PA: National Council of Teachers of English.

Simpson, M. K. (1986). A teacher's gift: Oral reading and the reading response journal. *Journal of Reading, 30*(1), 45–50.

Smith, F. (1982). *Writing and the writer*. Hillsdale, NJ: Erlbaum.

Smith, P. L., & Tompkins, G. E. (1988). Structured notetaking: A new strategy for content area readers. *Journal of Reading, 32*(1), 45–53.

Stauffer, R. G. (1970). *The language-experience approach to the teaching of reading*. New York: Harper & Row.

Stires, S. (1983). *Sentence combining: A composing book* (2nd ed.). New York: Random House.

Strong, W. (1986). *Creative approaches to sentence combining*. Urbana, IL: National Council of Teachers of English.

Temple, C., & Gillet, J. W. (1984). *Language arts: Learning processes and teaching practices*. Austin, TX: PRO-ED.

Wallace, G., Cohen, S. B., & Polloway, E. A. (1987). *Language arts: Teaching exceptional students*. Austin, TX: PRO-ED.

Wallace, G., & Kauffman, J. M. (1986). *Teaching students with learning and behavior problems* (3rd ed.). Columbus, OH: Merrill.

Whale, K. B., & Robinson, S. (1978). Modes of students' writing: A descriptive study. *Research in the Teaching of English, 12*, 349–355.

Whaley, J. F. (1981). Story grammars and reading instruction. *The Reading Teacher, 34*(8), 762–771.

Wiig, E. H., & Semel, E. M. (1984). *Language assessment and intervention for the learning disabled* (2nd ed.). Columbus, OH: Merrill.

Wixon, K., & Peters, C. (1985). How to do expository text mapping. *Reading Psychology, 6*, 169–179.

Wood, K. D. (1984). Probable passages: A writing strategy. *The Reading Teacher, 37*(6), 496–499.

Written Language Test Reviews

7

Laura Lyons Bailet

Quantification of written language proficiency can and should take many forms. No single test assesses comprehensively all aspects of written language achievement. Even if several standardized tests are administered, additional informal diagnostic activities are necessary to develop an appropriate remedial program. Fortunately, many standardized written language tests are available that provide psychologists and educators with a broad range of writing assessment instruments for identifying children who need special instruction.

Traditionally, writing tests have been dichotomized into atomistic tests, which measure individual writing skills such as spelling, grammar, and punctuation, and holistic measures, which evaluate the communicative effectiveness of a writing sample (Bain, 1988). Atomistic tests reflect a product approach to writing, whereas holistic assessment reflects the curricular and philosophical shift toward the process approach. The test format may be contrived, in which case the test provides the writing stimuli, such as a dictation spelling test, or spontaneous, in which the student composes a writing sample (Hammill & Larsen, 1996). Ideally, both atomistic and holistic assessment, employing both contrived and spontaneous formats, should be incorporated into a comprehensive evaluation of written language proficiency. Omission of any of these formats may result in failure to delineate thoroughly the nature of an individual's writing strengths and weaknesses.

At present, well-normed, reliable, and generally valid standardized tests are available that quantify dictation spelling skills, spontaneous spelling skills, vocabulary usage, syntactic accuracy, sentence combining ability, punctuation and capitalization usage, and written expressive skills. Whether measurement of these skills relates meaningfully to performance on typical classroom writing assignments is less certain (Bain, 1988; Hammill & Larsen, 1996). Even the spontaneous writing formats of some standardized tests may not relate sufficiently to classroom writing curricula. Many spontaneous writing tests employ pictures as a stimulus for writing creative stories, a format typically used in the classroom only for younger elementary students. Older students, in contrast, more often receive expository writing assignments. Performance on creative versus expository writing assignments often differs substantially. Thus, one must assess continuously the relevance of standardized data within the context of school-based written language experiences, requirements, and expectations.

The multifaceted nature of written expression makes objective, valid measurement difficult. The writing process may break down at the level of individual subskills, such as handwriting, punctuation, spelling, and grammar usage. On the other hand, for some individuals, the breakdown occurs only when all of these subskills must be integrated within the broader process of composing. The first goal of diagnosis, then, is to identify the most basic level at which a writing breakdown occurs, followed by identification of intervention strategies that facilitate more effective written communication. As Chapter 4 points out, particularly in the areas of syntax, cohesion, and coherence, no one has yet developed scoring methods that provide relevant, accurate standardized information.

Holistic assessment is a technique that, if used effectively, can preclude questions of relevance, because it is criterion referenced. This type of analysis assists the examiner in evaluating a student's ability to communicate ideas through writing. Its purpose is to avoid analyzing a composition in terms of mechanistic features. Rather, the composition's overall effectiveness in conveying ideas is assessed. This approach may enable teachers and students to maintain a more meaningful, interesting focus for writing activities, as opposed to spelling, grammar, and punctuation drills. Nonetheless, many individuals are unable to convey ideas well in writing because of significant difficulties with writing mechanics or subskills. For such individuals, both atomistic and holistic writing assessments contribute to understanding the nature and scope of written language deficits.

In reviewing standardized writing tests, two issues remained foremost in determining each test's usefulness. First, the technical characteristics were examined, including normative procedures and results of reliability and validity studies. Numerous texts describing the minimum standards necessary for adequate norming, reliability, and validity are available (e.g., Anastasi & Urbina, 1997; Salvia & Ysseldyke, 1991). In general, the technical quality of written language tests has improved significantly with the revision of older tests and development of new tests. Second, the specific issue of content validity was considered, in terms of representativeness of the writing sample collected, as well as the relevance of the data collected to the broader process of writing. Despite significant improvement in writing tests currently available, test users continue to have a major responsibility to review the technical characteristics of each test they administer, and also to reflect upon issues of test relevance for specific individuals and their educational or occupational milieus. No matter what standardized writing tests are administered, the diagnostician or teacher will need to devise informal assessment activities in order to program most effectively for each student.

The following reviews of tests are in alphabetical order by test name.

Boder Test of Reading–Spelling Patterns: A Diagnostic Screening Test for Subtypes of Reading Disability

Authors: S. Boder and S. Jarrico
Publisher: Psychological Corporation (1982)

Description

The *Boder Test of Reading–Spelling Patterns* is designed to identify specific reading disability subtypes by analyzing reading and spelling errors according to phonemic accuracy. It can be used with children from kindergarten through Grade 12, as well as with adults. Four possible subtypes of poor spellers are identified: (1) dysphonetics (fail to decode or spell words phonetically, but can read some words by sight method); (2) dyseidetics (make phonetically accurate errors in reading and spelling); (3) mixed dysphonetics–dyseidetics (have difficulty reading sight words and cannot read or spell phonetically); and (4) nonspecific reading disability (do not fit other categories).

The test consists of reading and spelling subtests. The reading subtest is administered first, with 1-second exposures per word to identify sight vocabulary. Words not read accurately during this portion are then presented untimed, to determine phonics skills.

The spelling subtest requires students to write from dictation both phonemically regular and irregular words from their sight reading vocabulary, as well as words they were unable to read. Directions for administration, particularly for the spelling portion, are complex, because each child writes different words, based on results from the reading subtest. Scoring procedures are well described but require considerable subjective judgment in terms of error classification.

Scores obtained include percentage of known words spelled correctly, percentage of unknown words spelled as good phonemic equivalents, and a reading quotient. This latter score is based on the concept of mental age, which has been shown to be unreliable.

Technical Characteristics

Normative Sample. This test was developed on the basis of the clinical performance of approximately 3,000 children. No demographic data on these children are provided.

Reliability. Test–retest reliability coefficients were calculated using very small sample sizes. The coefficients for the reading scores are within an acceptable range. For the spelling subtest, coefficients range from .56 to .89, many of which are below accepted standards for reliability.

Validity. Little validity information is provided. The authors cite unpublished research data from clinical studies reportedly verifying construct validity. However, this information, which is subjective, addresses clinical utility rather than objective construct validity. There is no objective information on which to determine content or criterion-related validity.

Critique

The *Boder Test of Reading–Spelling Patterns* can provide useful diagnostic information for understanding the nature of a child's reading and spelling disabilities, in that it assists the examiner in systematic analysis of error patterns. As compared with other standardized spelling tests, a strength of the *Boder Test of Reading–Spelling Patterns* is the shift in focus from spelling accuracy to examination of error patterns. However, the theoretical basis and diagnostic sensitivity of the test's error classification system has come under question in recent spelling literature. Because it examines only a few subskills that relate to reading and spelling, it does not provide a comprehensive diagnosis.

As a standardized reading and spelling measure, it is technically flawed particularly in the lack of information about the normative sample, low reliability coefficients, and the failure to provide objective validity data. Therefore, it should not be used for making school placement decisions or for program evaluation.

Group Writing Tests (GWT)

Authors: N. Mather and R. W. Woodcock
Publisher: Riverside (1997)

Description

The GWT is adapted from the *Woodcock–Johnson–Revised Tests of Achievement* (WJ–R) (Woodcock & Johnson, 1989) writing subtests and follows simi lar testing formats. All items for the GWT are new. The GWT is designed for use in schools and vocational situations for screening, program planning, and writing evaluation over time. The GWT is designed primarily for students in Grades 2 through college. Three levels are provided: Basic, for Grades 2 and 3; Intermediate, for Grades 4 to 7; and Advanced, for Grades 8 to college. The examiner can select a lower or higher level for a particular testing situation, to match the student's likely skill level. The GWT can be administered in one session or several. Total testing time takes approximately 1 hour for the whole battery. Four subtests are included: Dictation Spelling, Writing Samples, Editing, and Writing Fluency. These can be combined to yield three clusters: Total Writing, which includes all four subtests; Basic Writing Skills, which includes Dictation Spelling and Editing; and Expressive Writing Ability, which includes Writing Samples and Writing Fluency. Standard scores, percentiles, instructional zones, and age- and grade-equivalent scores can be derived. Scoring principles are similar to those in the WJ–R. Directions for scoring are detailed and clear. Nonetheless, the scoring of the Writing Samples and Writing Fluency subtests is time-consuming, particularly for groups of students.

Technical Characteristics

Normative Sample. The GWT was normed using the same sample as the WJ–R, described later in this chapter. The sample included 3,345 subjects ages 6 to 18 years, and 2,135 subjects ages 19 to greater than 90 years. The sample was stratified according to gender, race, ethnicity, geographic region, and community size. Additional factors of occupational status, years of education, and type of college attended were used to stratify the adult sample. Students with "severe handicaps" were excluded unless they attended regular education at least part time.

Reliability. Reliability for the GWT was calculated using the split-half procedure. Although most correlation coefficients were .85 or higher, on the Writing Fluency subtest, coefficients ranged from .59 to .87, with five out of eight reported coefficients falling less than .80. The standard errors of measurement (*SEM*s) on the Writing Fluency subtest also are large, ranging from 5.8 to 10 standard score points. The *SEM*s on the other subtests and clusters generally are 5 standard score points or less. The GWT does not provide information on test–retest or interscorer reliability.

Validity. Items selected for the GWT were modeled after items in the WJ–R. These items were rank-ordered by estimated difficulty and preliminary forms of the test were piloted. These results were then Rasch-calibrated and further adjusted to match the difficulty scale of the WJ–R comparable subtests. No information is provided to describe how the initial pool of items was selected. Some information is provided as a rationale for the GWT subtests and format. Results of several studies comparing GWT scores with scores from other writing tests indicated satisfactory concurrent validity.

Intercorrelations among GWT subtests and clusters indicated satisfactory construct validity.

Critique

The GWT provides a group format for testing several important writing skills. The normative sample meets accepted standards, although the exclusion of students in self-contained special education classrooms may be problematic, as they are likely to be assessed with this type of instrument. The GWT fails to give information on test–retest or interscorer reliability. Test–retest reliability data are particularly important when one uses test data to monitor student progress and evaluate programs, both of which are listed as intended uses of the GWT. Validity data are satisfactory, although additional explanation regarding item selection would be helpful. Scoring time and complexity may make the GWT impractical in most classroom situations. The GWT has merit as a screening instrument but should be used cautiously for other purposes.

Test of Adolescent and Adult Language—Third Edition (TOAL–3)

Authors: D. D. Hammill, V. L. Brown, S. C. Larsen, and J. L. Wiederholt
Publisher: PRO-ED (1994)

Description

The TOAL–3 is a measure of receptive and expressive oral and written language skills for individuals ages 12 through 24 years, 11 months. Eight subtests are included that measure vocabulary and grammar skills across the domains of listening, speaking, reading, and writing. Six subtests can be administered to groups, whereas the other two (the Speaking subtests) must be individually administered. For group administration, all students begin with Item 1 for each subtest. Testing is discontinued when the examiner feels that all students have obtained a ceiling of three incorrect responses out of five items. It is not clear how the examiner makes this determination in a group test situation. For individual testing, starting points by age are given in the manual. The two writing subtests, Writing/Vocabulary and Writing/ Grammar, measure ability to use given vocabulary words in sentences, and to combine two given sentences into one sentence. Administration procedures for these two subtests are generally clear. The manual specifies that the examiner cannot read the words to the student for the Writing/Vocabulary subtest; no such instruction is stated for the Writing/Grammar subtest. Examples of correct and incorrect responses are given for each test item. Raw scores are converted to scaled scores, composite quotients, and percentiles.

Technical Characteristics

Normative Sample. The TOAL–3 normative sample included 3,056 individuals. However, only data from 18- to 24-year-olds were collected in 1993 (587 subjects), whereas the remaining normative data were collected in 1980 and 1987 for earlier versions of this test. Subjects were drawn from 26 states and three Canadian provinces. Sex, race, ethnicity, residence, and geographic location characteristics of the norming sample were described by the authors as comparable to that of the general population. However, Richards (1998) criticized the normative methods as inadequate because few students were included from large city school systems. No information is provided to indicate whether students or young adults with disabilities were included in the normative sample.

Reliability. The authors report information pertaining to internal consistency, test–retest, and interscorer reliability. All internal consistency reliability coefficients meet or exceed .80. Particularly for the composite quotients, the content reliability coefficients are consistently .90 or higher. A test–retest study of 59 college students using the TOAL–3 indicated correlation coefficients of .83 and .79 on the Writing/Vocabulary and Writing/Grammar subtests, respectively, and .87 on the Writing Composite score.

For the three subtests that require subjective judgment, the authors conducted a study of interscorer reliability on the TOAL, using a sample of 15 protocols from ninth graders. Mean coefficients of .87 for Writing/Vocabulary and .98 for Writing/Grammar indicate that scoring procedures are sufficient for scorer consistency.

Validity. Information related to content, criterion-related, and construct validity is presented. Analyses of internal consistency and discussion of the choice of test format establish the content validity of the TOAL–3 subtests. Several studies of criterion validity were reported that involved the TOAL, TOAL–2, and TOAL–3. Results indicated that scores from these measures were strongly correlated with scores from several other oral language, reading, and written language tests. One study also showed that the TOAL–3 correctly identified 89% of 28 subjects with language learning disabilities and 86% of 28 subjects without language learning disabilities.

Several studies were undertaken to assess construct validity. The authors examined the change in subtest means and standard deviations across the age range in the normative sample. Changes in raw scores on the writing subtests are of very low magnitude, typically spanning only 5 points from age 12 years to 24 years, with standard deviations ranging from 3 to 10 points. Correlations of test scores with age are low to very low for 12- to 16-year-olds, and very low to nonexistent for 17- to 24-year-olds. It is not clear how this data supports the authors' claim of construct validity.

The authors correlated TOAL scores with scores from the *California Short-Form Test of Academic Aptitude*, for a sample of 32 children, with a resultant coefficient of .79. However, this intelligence test dates from 1973 and thus has outdated norms. Several studies are cited that found lower TOAL and TOAL–3 scores for children with learning disabilities, mental retardation, and poor reading skills, as well as juvenile delinquents. Factor analyses and item validity studies also are reported as evidence of construct validity.

Critique

The TOAL–3 has outdated norms for subjects ages 12 through 17 years, and the normative sample may not be completely representative of the students who are likely to be administered the test. Reliability appears satisfactory. Many of the validity studies were conducted using the original TOAL and other outdated tests; others do not definitively demonstrate the validity issue in question. From a practical standpoint, the writing subtests involve reading, which may confound results for individual students. The TOAL–3 writing subtests therefore are not recommended as primary measures of writing skills for diagnosis, placement, or research purposes.

Test of Early Written Language—Second Edition (TEWL–2)

Authors: W. P. Hresko, S. R. Herron, and P. K. Peak
Publisher: PRO-ED (1996)

Description

The TEWL–2 was designed to measure prewriting and writing skills of children ages 3 years to 10 years, 11 months. The norms for children under age 4 years were provided for research purposes only. The TEWL–2 should not be administered for clinical or educational purposes to children less than 4 years of age. It was designed to identify children with significant delays in early writing skills and to determine an individual child's writing strengths and weaknesses. The authors state that the TEWL–2 can be used to measure writing progress relative to special intervention, and for research. As compared with the TEWL, the age range has been extended, the total number of items has increased, and two forms (A and B) have been developed.

The TEWL-2 consists of the Basic Writing subtest, which assesses mechanical aspects of writing, and the Contextual Writing subtest, which measures ability to produce a writing sample. For each subtest, age equivalent scores, normal curve equivalent (NCE) scores, percentiles, and quotients can be derived. The two subtest scores can be combined to yield a Global Writing Quotient. Administration time is 30 to 45 minutes. The Basic Writing subtest should be administered to individuals, as basals and ceilings must be obtained. The starting point varies according to the child's age. The Contextual Writing subtest may be administered to individuals or groups and does not involve basals or ceilings.

The Basic Writing subtest measures knowledge and skills related to writing purposes, drawing, writing vocabulary (e.g., *pencil, cursive, newspaper, sentence*), spelling, punctuation, sentence combining, and sentence logic. Scoring criteria are provided for each item and generally are clear. A picture prompt is provided for the Contextual Writing subtest, one for children ages 5 years to 6 years, 11 months, and another for older children. Writing samples are scored according to 14 criteria that measure inclusion of a theme, plot sequence, descriptive details, characters, dialogue, elaboration beyond the picture, spelling, and sentence structure. Scores for each criterion range from zero to 3, and descriptions are provided for each score. An expanded scoring guide is included in the test kit, which contains 10 writing samples and an explanation of appropriate scoring for each criterion.

Technical Characteristics

Normative Sample. A new standardization sample of 1,479 children was obtained for the TEWL-2. Characteristics relative to age, race, ethnicity, gender, urban /rural residence, and geographic region are provided and generally conform to 1990 U.S. census data. Children known to have learning disabilities, speech–language disorder, or mental retardation were included in the standardization sample with representative frequency.

Reliability. In an internal consistency study, all coefficient alphas were at or above .90. *SEM*s ranged from 1.5 to 3.7 for standard scores on the Basic Writing subtest, and from 4.2 to 4.7 for standard scores on the Contextual Writing subtest. Four test–retest and alternate form studies were conducted with time intervals varying from 14 to 21 days. Reliability coefficients all were above .80 for each of the two subtests, and above .90 for the Global Writing quotient. Interscorer reliability coefficients ranged from .92 to .99 when six scorers scored 25 randomly selected tests from the normative sample.

Validity. To address content validity, the authors describe existing literature on skills that subserve writing development and the process used to
identify appropriate test items. Item discrimination, difficulty, and potential
cultural bias were analyzed, and items not meeting specified criteria were
modified or eliminated (Hurford, 1998). Several concurrent validity studies
were conducted comparing scores on the TEWL–2 with scores on other academic achievement tests for samples of students attending public or private
schools in Texas. Results generally reflected satisfactory concurrent validity.
A predictive validity study with the TEWL indicated that students who had
performed poorly tended to remain below average in writing several years
later, whereas those who had performed average or above were continuing to
do so. This study appears to have been based on teacher judgment of current
writing ability, although this was not clearly specified. Scores for 40 students
on the TEWL, administered in the fall of 1993, were correlated with their
scores on the TEWL–2 during standardization, with a resultant coefficient of
.62. Construct validity was assessed by correlating TEWL–2 scores with
scores on several cognitive measures. Coefficients ranged from .31 to .71, and
all were statistically significant. Mean scores on the TEWL–2 for several
groups of students receiving special education were significantly below average. Means and standard deviations were provided for each age interval in
the normative sample and showed linear growth, as would be expected.

Critique

The TEWL–2 represents a significant improvement over the TEWL and provides a reliable, valid, and clinically useful tool to assess writing ability in
young children. The addition of test items and the writing sample expand the
scope and meaningfulness of this test. Extensive reliability and validity studies indicate the test authors' willingness to address previous criticisms of the
TEWL (Trevisan, 1998). Additional studies of the TEWL–2's sensitivity and
specificity would be useful in determining its accuracy in identifying young
children with writing deficits in need of special intervention.

Test of Phonological Awareness (TOPA)

Authors: J. K. Torgesen and B. R. Bryant
Publisher: PRO-ED (1994)

Description

The TOPA is not a writing test. Rather, it measures phonological awareness
skills, which have been shown through extensive empirical research to sub

Written Language Test Reviews ⟶ 231

serve the development of reading and spelling skills. It is included in this chapter because I believe that comprehensive assessment of a student's writing problems may need to incorporate measures of phonological awareness. Its stated primary purpose is to identify early students who require special training in phonological awareness. It is also recommended as part of a larger screening battery for children in the early elementary grades, and for research. The TOPA has two forms: a kindergarten version designed for students in the latter half of their kindergarten year, and an early elementary version for students in first and second grades. It can be administered individually or in groups. Each version consists of two parts, each containing 10 items. Students mark a picture-based answer form in response to items presented orally by the examiner. At the kindergarten level, students compare beginning consonant sounds in single-syllable words. For the early elementary level, students compare ending consonant sounds in single-syllable words. The test takes approximately 10 minutes to administer. Instructions are clear and easy to follow. Test responses are scored as correct or incorrect. Raw scores are converted to percentiles, and several types of standard scores, including W-scores, stanines, quotients, T-scores, z-scores, and normal curve equivalents.

Technical Characteristics

Normative Sample. The kindergarten version of the TOPA was normed on 857 students in 10 states. The early elementary version was normed on 3,654 students in 38 states. The sample is described according to age, gender, race, ethnicity, place of residence, and geographical region and is consistent with 1990 census data. No information is given to indicate whether students in special education were included.

Reliability. Internal consistency coefficients by age ranged from .87 to .91. Test–retest reliability was assessed with 40 kindergarten and 69 first-grade students, with a time interval of 6 and 8 weeks, respectively. After statistically removing the error associated with internal consistency, the test–retest coefficient was .94 for kindergarten, and .77 for first grade. This latter value is unacceptably low for test–retest reliability. The author explained that the longer time interval and ongoing reading instruction were likely factors contributing to score instability at the first-grade level. This finding deserves further investigation. The *SEM*s range from 4.5 to 5.4 points for the summary quotient.

Validity. Extensive discussion is devoted to validity issues for the TOPA, including a lengthy description of several types of phonological tasks and their relationships with one another. The literature review, Torgesen's own extensive research on phonological awareness skills, and item discrimination and item difficulty analyses indicate adequate content and construct validity. Concurrent validity was established by correlating TOPA scores with scores on other phonological awareness tasks, experimental measures of invented spelling ability, and standardized early reading measures. Predictive validity was established by correlating TOPA scores in kindergarten with standardized reading scores at the end of first grade. The correlation coefficient was .62, such that between 30% and 40% of the variance in reading scores was accounted for by the TOPA scores from the previous year.

Critique

The TOPA fills a critical need in providing a standardized measure of phonological awareness skills in young children. The normative procedures are adequate, and validity information is excellent. The relatively low test–retest reliability coefficient for the early elementary version is somewhat troublesome and should be studied further. Nonetheless, this test marks a significant advance in our ability to measure early phonological awareness skills that contribute to reading and spelling development.

Test of Written Expression (TOWE)

Authors: R. McGhee, B. R. Bryant, S. C. Larsen, and D. M. Rivera
Publisher: PRO-ED (1995)

Description

The TOWE is a writing test for students ages 6 years, 6 months through 14 years, 11 months. It consists of two parts: a section of individual test items assessing alphabet letter-writing skill, capitalization, punctuation, spelling, ideation, semantics, and syntax, and an essay written in response to a story starter. The written story is administered only to students age 8 and above. It is scored on length, presence of paragraphs, plot sequence, descriptive details, spelling, and grammatical accuracy. The test can be administered to groups or individuals. Various starting points are specified according to the students' grade level. For students tested in a group who fail to obtain a basal of five consecutive, correct responses, and a ceiling of five consecutive incorrect responses, testing must be completed individually. Raw scores are converted to standard scores, percentiles, and grade equivalents.

    Administration instructions for individual test items and the essay are generally clear. The manual does not state whether instructions can be repeated or explained, which may cause problems for some students. Responses are marked in a booklet, which is visually confusing for Items 1 through 19. These items are not consistently arranged in consecutive order, either from left to right or top to bottom. Particularly when administered to groups of young students, one could envision that answers would be marked in the wrong places, or students could become confused and lost. For example, Item 14 is at the bottom of page 1 in the student booklet, followed by Item 13 at the top of page 2 (Perlman, 1998). In addition, for Items 9 and 18, the student is required to give an oral response, yet there is no indication in the manual as to how this is accomplished in a group test situation. Scoring instructions for individual items in the first part of the test are usually clear. However, no samples are given, and grammar terms, such as *dependent clause*, upon which scoring is based, are not defined. For the essay, scoring criteria are clearly described, and several scored samples are provided in the test manual.

Technical Characteristics

Normative Sample. The TOWE was normed on 1,355 students from 21 states. Information on gender, residence, race, ethnicity, and geographic area are provided and compare favorably to 1990 U.S. census data. However, no information is given on socioeconomic status or whether students with disabilities were included in the normative process. Samples for each age group are small, particularly for 6-year-olds ($n = 81$) and 14-year-olds ($n = 87$) (Perlman, 1998).

Reliability. Internal consistency was determined using coefficient alphas for each 1-year age interval. For the individual items portion of the TOWE, these coefficients averaged .92 and ranged from .88 to .95. For the essay, the average was .90, with coefficients ranging from .78 to .93. The lowest coefficients occurred for the youngest subjects in the normative sample. Interscorer reliability was assessed by having two individuals score 30 protocols, resulting in correlation coefficients of .98 for the individual items portion, and .89 for the essay. Test–retest reliability was assessed by administering the TOWE twice to 26 children, using a 2-week test interval. Results indicated coefficients of .83 and .99 for the two portions of the TOWE, after variance attributable to internal consistency and interscorer reliability was extracted.

Validity. The authors describe in detail their efforts to identify test items with satisfactory content validity. They examined numerous published language arts programs and teacher activities to select an initial group of 100 items. These items were then piloted with small numbers of students at several age levels. They also computed item discrimination and item difficulty using the point biserial correlation technique. These correlations were quite low at age 6 years for the individual items portion of the TOWE (median = .00 for both item discrimination and item difficulty) and at age 8 years for the essay (median = .15 for item discrimination and .04 for item difficulty). Values were higher and thus more acceptable for older students. Several concurrent validity studies were undertaken comparing TOWE scores to scores from several other writing tests. Correlation coefficients indicated adequate concurrent validity. Several types of construct validity studies revealed adequate correlation with measures of general cognitive ability and other academic achievement areas such as reading, and ability to differentiate students by age and writing ability. Two studies indicated no evidence of potential racial bias in the TOWE.

Critique

The TOWE is an interesting measure of writing ability with some strengths as well as several significant weaknesses. Its major strength is the use of an interesting story starter to elicit an essay. Inconsistencies in the student response booklet and examiner instructions for administering and scoring individual items may cause significant practical problems in use of the TOWE. Technical data provided in the manual suggest that it lacks sufficient item discrimination and reliability for students ages 6 through 8 years. The normative sample is small, and essential information on socioeconomic status and inclusion of students with disabilities is not provided. Users are cautioned not to rely exclusively on the TOWE for assessing a student's writing skills.

Test of Written Language—Third Edition (TOWL-3)

Authors: D. D. Hammill and S. C. Larsen
Publisher: PRO-ED (1996)

Description

The TOWL-3 is designed to measure conventional (i.e., spelling, punctuation, and capitalization), linguistic (i.e., semantic and syntactic), and cognitive components of written language production for individuals ages 7 years through 17 years, 11 months. It includes five contrived subtests measuring written vocabulary usage, sentence dictation spelling, sentence dictation punctuation and capitalization, ability to correct illogical sentences, and sentence combining. In addition, the student is asked to generate a story from a picture prompt, from which scores for three spontaneous subtests are obtained: Contextual Conventions, Contextual Language, and Story Construction. The TOWL-3 thus has been shortened to 8 subtests, as compared to 10 for the TOWL-2. This test is designed primarily for individual administration, although it can be given to groups and special instructions are provided for this. The TOWL-3 takes approximately 90 minutes to administer in its entirety. Administration and scoring procedures are clearly written and easy to follow; nonetheless, scoring of the spontaneous writing sample is moderately complex and time-consuming. Scores include subtest standard scores and percentiles, and quotients for composite scores. Age and grade equivalent scores also are provided.

Technical Characteristics

Normative Sample. The TOWL–3 normative sample consisted of 2,217 students from 25 states. An entirely new norming sample was drawn for the TOWL–3. The sample is described with respect to sex, place of residence, race, age, ethnicity, geographic area, family income, educational level of parents, and disabling condition. Ten percent of the normative sample had a learning disability, speech–language disorder, or mental handicap. Comparison of the normative sample characteristics with census information indicates that it represents accurately the general school-age population.

Reliability. The test authors provide information related to internal consistency, alternate form, test–retest, and interscorer reliability. The coefficient alpha method was used to assess internal consistency. Average coefficients for the entire normative sample were greater than .80 for all subtests except Contextual Conventions (.70). For the three composite scales, average coefficients ranged from .91 to .97. The authors also calculated coefficients for selected subgroups according to gender, ethnicity, and disability status.

Alternate form reliability studies indicated coefficients generally above .80, except for the Contextual Conventions subtest (.71). Composite means and standard deviations for Forms A and B are almost the same for all age levels. Test–retest reliability was assessed by administering both forms of the TOWL–3 to 27 second graders and 28 twelfth graders twice, with a 2-week time interval between test sessions. Reliability coefficients ranged from .72 to .93, with averages falling between .75 and .89. The lowest coefficients occurred on the Style, Contextual Conventions, Contextual Language, and Story Construction subtests. These values suggest some degree of score instability, at least for the youngest and oldest students for whom the TOWL–3 was designed.

Interscorer reliability was assessed using 38 response protocols, each scored by two PRO-ED staff members familiar with the scoring procedures. Coefficients for the subtests ranged from .80 to .97. For the three composite scores, all coefficients were >.90. Given the relative complexity of scoring the spontaneous writing sample, a study involving scorers less familiar with the development of the TOWL–3 would be beneficial.

Validity. Information pertaining to content, criterion-related, and construct validity is presented in the TOWL–3 manual. Extensive discussion of test rationale and statistical item analysis indicate adequate content validity for students ages 9 years and above. However, for students 7 to 8 years of age, the median discrimination indices are too low for the Contrived subtests, such that the TOWL–3 may have little utility for that age group (Bucy, 1998; Hansen, 1998).

To examine criterion-related validity, TOWL–3 scores of 76 elementary school students were correlated with scores on the Writing Scale of the *Comprehensive Scales of Student Abilities* (Hammil & Hresko, 1994), a teacher rating scale that assesses multiple school performance skills. All coefficients were statistically significant at $p < .05$ and were in the range of .50, indicating moderate correlation. There were some differences in degree of correlation for subtests within Form A versus Form B, with higher correlations occurring for Form B.

Extensive studies relating to construct validity are reported in the TOWL–3 manual. The authors report coefficients between TOWL–3 scores and chronological age. Mean raw scores and standard deviations for each age level in the standardization sample are provided and show expected score increases from age 7 to 14 years on most subtests, at which point the scores remain essentially the same to age 17 years. However, on the Contextual Conventions and Story Construction subtests, mean scores remain static from age 11 to 17 years. Correlations with age are not significant at this age level. This indicates that the TOWL–3 lacks discriminatory power in identifying older students with more subtle writing deficits. Factor analyses, studies of group differentiation, and correlations with intelligence and achievement measures generally reflect adequate construct validity.

Critique

The TOWL–3 provides a comprehensive measure of many skills critical to written expression proficiency. Normative procedures appear adequate. Test–retest reliability coefficients are not consistently high enough across all subtests and age levels, and additional interscorer reliability studies are needed due to the complexity and subjectivity of scoring procedures. Some validity studies reveal potential problems in test construction and content for both young elementary students and students age 13 years and above.

Administration time is excessively long for some students with significant writing difficulties, although considerable information can be gained. My own experience is that the scoring procedures for the writing sample often yield average scores, even on stories that are clearly deficient in many ways. The educational utility of the TOWL–3 thus remains in question despite some adequate technical characteristics.

Test of Written Spelling—Fourth Edition (TWS-4)

Authors: S. C. Larsen, D. D. Hammill, and L. Moats
Publisher: PRO-ED (1999)

Description

The TWS–4 is a single-word dictation spelling test for individuals ages 6 years to 18 years, 11 months. It can be administered to individuals or groups. Two forms, A and B, are now available. The TWS–4 consists of the same words used in the TWS–3. However, instead of Predictable and Unpredictable word subtests, these were combined and then split into the two alternate forms. The stated purposes of the test are for identification of a learning disorder, documentation of spelling progress, and research. The authors explicitly state that the TWS–4 does not provide enough detailed information to be used as the basis for instructional planning. A nice addition to the manual is a section describing supplementary diagnostic activities that are helpful for this purpose.

Administration and scoring procedures are well presented and easy to follow. The student writes a response for each dictated word. Recommended starting points for various age levels are provided. Testing is terminated after the child makes five consecutive errors. All responses are scored as correct or incorrect. A single raw score is converted to percentiles, standard scores, and age and grade equivalents.

Technical Characteristics

Normative Sample. The TWS–4 was not renormed. The normative sample included 4,097 children tested in 1986 and 855 children tested in 1993 for the TWS–2, yielding a combined normative sample of 4,952. Subjects were selected from 23 states. Demographic characteristics including sex, place of residence, race, ethnic identity, and age are provided and conform satisfactorily to national demographic data. The authors did not state whether individuals with disabilities were included in the norming sample.

Reliability. Internal consistency reliability was computed using Cronbach's coefficient alpha method. Nearly all coefficients were greater than .90. *SEM*s ranged from 3 to 5 standard score points. Alternate form reliability coefficients were above .90 except at age 6 ($r = .86$). The authors reported coefficients greater than .90 for test–retest reliability on both forms of the TWS–4, using a sample of 41 students in Grades 1, 3, and 6 with a 2-week interval between test administrations. Interscorer reliability was .99, which reflects the clear administration procedures and scoring ease for the TWS–4. These high coefficients across a variety of reliability studies suggest excellent reliability for the TWS–4.

Validity. Extensive information is provided concerning item selection and item analysis for the original TWS. Items were included only if they appeared in 10 basal spelling series for Grades 1 through 8. For high school level items, the authors consulted the *EDL Core Vocabularies in Reading, Mathematics, Science, and Social Studies* (Taylor et al., 1979). For the TWS–4, the authors verified that all words in the test still occurred with high frequency in leading basal spelling series and the current EDL list. Extensive item discrimination, item difficulty, and item bias statistical analyses also were conducted for the TWS–4, and no problems with test content were identified. The content validity of the TWS–4 thus remains strong.

The authors report concurrent validity studies for the original TWS, using four other standardized measures of spelling ability. Coefficients ranged from .78 to .97, thus falling within acceptable limits. Two recent studies with the TWS–4 also demonstrated moderate concurrent validity with other spelling tests and teachers' ratings of students' spelling ability. In terms of construct validity, the authors note that raw scores among the normative sample increase as expected on the basis of normal development. Studies are cited that indicate moderate degrees of correlation between TWS–4 scores and scores on several achievement and aptitude tests.

Critique

The TWS–4 is a technically sound standardized measure of spelling achievement that provides a broad sample of a child's dictation spelling skills. The authors responded well to previous criticisms of the TWS, TWS–2, and TWS–3 by eliminating the Predictable and Unpredictable Words subtests. They also added excellent descriptions of spelling development and supplementary diagnostic activities for children with spelling problems. Numerous additional reliability and validity studies were undertaken with the TWS–4, and their results reflect a technically strong product. The TWS–4 is highly recommended as the dictation spelling test of choice for identification of students with spelling disabilities, documentation of progress, and research.

Wechsler Individual Achievement Test (WIAT)

Author: Psychological Corporation
Publisher: Psychological Corporation (1992)

Description

The WIAT is an individually administered achievement test designed for students ages 5 years through 19 years, 11 months, or students in Kindergarten through Grade 12. It was co-normed with the *Wechsler Intelligence Scale for Children–Third Edition* (Wechsler, 1991) to provide a more precise means of identifying discrepancies between achievement and intelligence. The WIAT includes subtests measuring reading, mathematics, spelling, written expression, listening comprehension, and oral expression. A screening battery that includes the Basic Reading, Mathematics Reasoning, and Spelling subtests can be administered in 10 to 15 minutes. The complete battery takes approximately 30 to 50 minutes for younger students, and 1 hour for older students. Various starting points are indicated in the manual according to the student's grade in school. The focus of this review will be on the Spelling and Written Expression subtests.

The WIAT Spelling subtest measures ability to write letters when either the letter name or letter sound is dictated, and to write words to dictation. Responses are scored as correct or incorrect. The Written Expression subtest is administered only to children in Grade 3 or above, and is recommended only for children who score more than 15 items correct on the Spelling subtest. However, the examiner's judgment is allowed in determining whether to administer the Written Expression subtest to a poor speller. Two writing prompts are provided. The first is to be used on first administration and the second for retesting. For each, the student is instructed to write a letter on a particular topic. The student is told that spelling errors will not be marked and that the address, salutation, and closing do not have to be included. Scoring is based on a Likert-type scale, with ratings from 1 to 4 for six different writing elements. A holistic scoring method also is available, although standard scores cannot be generated with this method. For each subtest and composite scale, standard scores, percentiles, NCEs, stanines, and age and grade equivalents can be derived. Two different methods for determining discrepancies between academic achievement and intelligence are provided, including the predicted-achievement and simple-difference methods.

Technical Characteristics

Normative Sample. The WIAT normative sample included 4,252 children attending kindergarten through Grade 12. The sample included approximately equal numbers of males and females. Proportions of children from various races and ethnic groups were generally comparable to 1988 U.S. census data, although case weighting was employed to make some adjustments. Subjects were drawn from the four major geographic regions in the U.S. and were stratified according to parent education categories. Both public and private schools were included. Students with various handicapping conditions who were receiving mainstream special services were included in the sample. A subset of the WIAT standardization sample, consisting of 1,284 children, also were administered the WISC–3.

Reliability. Internal consistency was assessed using the split-half method, and coefficients generally are acceptable. They range from .80 to .93 across age groups for the Spelling subtest, and from .76 to .84 for the Written Expression subtest. *SEM*s average 4.96 on Spelling and 6.59 on Written Expression. Test–retest reliability was assessed with a sample of 367 children across five grades, tested twice within a time interval ranging from 12 to 52 days. For Spelling, the average coefficient across the five grades was .94, whereas for Written Expression, the average was .77. For the Writing composite, the average coefficient was .94. A study assessing interscorer reliability on the Written Expression subtest yielded coefficients of .89 for Prompt 1 and .79 for Prompt 2. A lengthy description and several tables are devoted to demonstrating how to determine the statistical significance of intersubtest scatter, and the reliability of these score differences.

Validity. The WIAT authors used both expert judgment and empirical item analysis to ensure content validity. The seven achievement areas listed in Public Law 94-142 (Education for All Handicapped Children Act of 1975) were included in the WIAT, and multiple sources were used to identify the scope and item content for each subtest. Rasch analyses were conducted to assess item difficulty. Potential item bias was assessed statistically and by a panel of experienced item reviewers. Construct validity was addressed through discussion of patterns of intercorrelations among WIAT subtests, and through correlational analyses with the Wechsler intelligence scales. Numerous studies comparing WIAT scores with scores on other achievement measures, school grades, and diagnosed special education classifications are described and provide extensive criterion-related validity evidence.

Critique

The WIAT represents a technically superior measure of academic achievement, particularly given the ability to calculate the significance of ability–achievement discrepancies using scores from the Wechsler intelligence tests. Administration and scoring procedures are well written, although scoring of the Written Expression subtest takes considerable time and effort. This test is strongly recommended for identifying children with possible learning disabilities.

Wide Range Achievement Test—3 (WRAT—3)

Author: G. S. Wilkinson
Publisher: Wide Range, Inc. (1993)

Description

The WRAT–3 is a short academic achievement test that includes measures of spelling, reading, and mathematics for individuals ages 5 to 75. Two forms are available, the Blue and Tan forms. There are no longer two separate levels of this test. The focus of this review will be the Spelling subtest.

The Spelling subtest follows a single-word dictation format requiring written responses. A prespelling section also can be administered, which includes writing one's name and writing dictated alphabet letters. All subjects begin with the first spelling item and continue until they misspell 10 consecutive words. All responses are scored as correct or incorrect. Scores are converted to standard scores, percentiles, and grade equivalents.

Technical Characteristics

Normative Sample. The normative sample consisted of 4,433 individuals across 23 age groups. A stratified national sample was selected on a random basis, controlling for age, sex, ethnicity, geographical region, and socioeconomic status. Students in special education were included in the normative sample if they were able to complete the test under standard conditions. All normative subjects took both forms of the WRAT–3 at the same test session. Subjects were tested individually for the Reading subtest, and in groups for the Spelling and Arithmetic subtests.

Reliability. The authors report coefficients ranging from .83 to .95 for measures of internal consistency on the Spelling subtest. Test–retest reliability coefficients ranging from .93 to .96 on the Spelling subtest were obtained, using a sample of 142 subjects. Alternate form correlations averaged .93 for the Spelling subtest. *SEM*s for standard scores ranged from 3.4 for the oldest subjects to 6.2 for 8-year-olds. Average *SEM*s for the Blue and Tan versions were 4.8 and 4.9, respectively.

Validity. The authors discuss issues of content, construct, and concurrent validity in the test manual. Rasch analysis was employed to ensure a broad range of item difficulty. However, many of the test items in the WRAT–3 were first developed in the original WRAT, dating as far back as 1936. No compelling evidence is provided to demonstrate that test content is appropriate according to current prevailing standards. The WRAT–3 includes a letter-writing section for young children, which reflects an improvement over the figure-copying task in the WRAT–R. Mabry (1995) and A. W. Ward (1995) have criticized the WRAT–3 for a lack of substantive information pertaining to construct validity.

Several concurrent validity studies for the WRAT–3 are reported, comparing WRAT–3 scores with scores on other standardized achievement measures. Correlation coefficients are in the acceptable range for these studies. The author also reports data from several studies assessing the WRAT– 3's ability to discriminate between children in special education and a matched control sample from the normative pool. The WRAT–3 was fairly accurate in identifying the students in special education, but it correctly classified only 56% of students from the normative sample.

Critique

The WRAT–3 represents a revision of an academic achievement screening test that has been used for many decades. The normative procedures and reliability studies appear generally adequate, although the *SEM*s for young children are quite large. Content and construct validity information is inadequate. The WRAT–3 Spelling subtest thus should not be used as a primary instrument for identifying students with spelling disability.

Woodcock—Johnson—Revised Tests of Achievement (Written Language Cluster)

Authors: R. W. Woodcock and M. B. Johnson
Publisher: Riverside Publishing (1989)

Description

The *Woodcock–Johnson Psycho-Educational Battery–Revised* (WJ–R), Tests of Achievement, is part of a larger battery that includes measures of cognitive ability. The entire battery is designed for individuals ages 2 through 90-plus years and is individually administered. There are two comparable forms of the WJ–R achievement battery, Forms A and B. Subtests are divided into the Standard Battery and Supplemental Battery. The writing subtests will be the primary focus of this review: Dictation, Writing Samples, Proofing, Writing Fluency, Punctuation and Capitalization, Spelling, Usage, and Handwriting. Review of some technical characteristics pertains to the battery as a whole.

The WJ–R Broad Written Language Cluster consists of the Dictation and Writing Samples subtests, both of which are included in the Standard Battery. The Dictation subtest includes items requiring the subject to copy marks, mark a line or circle within boundaries, and write alphabet letters, words, abbreviations, and punctuation marks from dictation. Several items assess knowledge of regular and irregular plural forms. The Writing Samples subtest requires the child to either complete a sentence with a written response, or generate a complete sentence in response to a picture and verbal instruction from the examiner.

The other writing subtests are part of the Supplemental Battery. The Proofing subtest requires the student to read sentences and identify errors in word usage, spelling, punctuation, and capitalization. The Writing Fluency subtest provides a picture stimulus and several words with which the student must quickly write a sentence. The Punctuation and Capitalization, Spelling, and Usage subtests are scored based on responses within the Dictation and Proofing subtests. The Handwriting subtest score is obtained by comparing the child's handwriting in the Writing Samples subtest with a ranked scale of handwriting samples in the test manual. The Dictation and Proofing subtest scores can be combined to yield a Basic Writing Skills cluster. The Writing Samples and Writing Fluency subtests combined yield a Written Expression cluster. Administration and scoring procedures are clearly presented and easy to follow. Scoring criteria for the Writing Samples subtest are somewhat subjective and time-consuming, although numerous examples of correct and incorrect responses are provided. Raw scores can be converted to age and grade equivalent scores, percentiles, standard scores, stanines, and normal curve equivalent scores. Scoring is time-consuming, as it is a multistep process involving calculations and the use of several tables. A computer scoring program is available.

Technical Characteristics

Normative Sample. The normative sample included 705 children ages 2 to 5 years and not enrolled in kindergarten, 3,245 students in Kindergarten through Grade 12, 916 individuals in colleges or universities, and 1,493 individuals age 14 to greater than 90 years who were not enrolled in school, for a total of 6,359 subjects. It is not clear why or how adolescent subjects not enrolled in school were included in the norming sample. Normative data were gathered from 1986 to 1988. Sex, race, ethnicity, geographic location, place of residence, and several indices of socioeconomic status were used to obtain a representative sample comparable to U.S. census data. Students with severe handicaps were not included in the normative sample unless they were enrolled at least part time in regular education.

Reliability. Numerous types of reliability studies are described in an extensive technical manual (McGrew, Werder, & Woodcock, 1991). Internal consistency coefficients generally exceeded .80, and most cluster coefficients exceeded .90. Test–retest coefficients were available on only some of the writing subtests and ranged from .80 to .91. The Writing Samples and Writing Fluency subtests were not included. Several studies of interrater reliability were described for the Writing Samples, Writing Fluency, and Handwriting subtests. Correlation coefficients were mostly above .90 for Writing Samples and Writing Fluency but ranged from .71 to .85 for Handwriting.

Validity. The WJ–R authors describe content validity in the technical manual but provide little specific information on how items were selected or statistical analyses to demonstrate objective evidence of content validity. The Dictation subtest includes many items that typically do not appear in other dictation tests and also yields a very small sample of responses for each of the skills assessed (e.g., spelling, grammar, punctuation, capitalization). Several concurrent validity studies are described for the WJ–R writing subtests and other standardized writing tests. Correlation coefficients are generally acceptable. Construct validity was assessed by examining patterns of intercorrelations among subtests and conducting factor analyses. The authors also cite studies demonstrating that WJ–R scores accurately differentiate gifted students, normal students, students with learning disabilities, and students with mental retardation.

Critique

The WJ–R clearly has become one of the major academic achievement measures used nationwide to determine eligibility for special education programs and document academic progress for individual students. The normative procedure is technically sound. Reliability and validity data are generally adequate. The content and format of some of the WJ–R writing subtests offer unique types of writing assessment, although the small number of items to measure spelling, punctuation, and capitalization limits their diagnostic utility. Many teachers and counselors find the scoring of Writing Samples too time-consuming, such that writing assessment is often limited to dictation spelling and proofreading skills. Additional formal and informal measures should be administered with the WJ–R to obtain a more representative picture of a student's current writing skills and instructional needs, and to determine eligibility for special education services.

Writing Process Test (WPT)

Authors: R. Warden and T. A. Hutchinson
Publisher: Riverside (1992)

Description

The WPT is designed to measure written expression skills in a manner that reflects the cognitive-process model. It can be administered individually or in groups for students in Grades 2 through 12. There are two alternate forms, A and B, each of which requires the student to write a composition on a given topic. The test is administered in two parts. For the first part, the student is instructed to plan and write a composition within 45 minutes. The student is then asked to respond to questions regarding his or her use of specific strategies during the writing process, and to evaluate the composition's effectiveness in relation to specific criteria. After at least 1 day, the child is asked to edit the first draft and complete another questionnaire regarding the use of revision strategies.

The writing samples are scored for 10 features using a 5-point scale. These features are clustered into two categories: Development, which includes purpose, audience, vocabulary, style, and organization; and Fluency, which includes sentence structure, grammar usage, punctuation, and spelling. Ratings from each scale can be summed to produce a total score that converts to a percentile rank or standard score. Percentiles are available by age and grade. Percentiles and standard scores can be obtained for both the rater's and writer's scores for a writing sample. Directions for test administration and scoring are clear and comprehensive. The authors have provided numerous supports for learning to score the WPT, including a training video, group training procedures, and calibration samples.

Technical Characteristics

Normative Sample. The WPT was normed on 4,286 students in Grades 2 through 12 in 11 school districts across the United States. A subset of 571 students was administered both Forms A and B. More students per grade were included for elementary and intermediate levels than for the high school level. The sample is described with respect to geographic region, sex, race, and school district size, and 122 participants identified themselves as being of Spanish origin. No information is provided on socioeconomic status of participants, and schools from the Northeast are overrepresented, whereas the South is underrepresented.

Reliability. Information is provided on internal consistency, interrater agreement, intrarater consistency, and alternate form reliability. Coefficients for the internal consistency of raters' scores range from .77 to .89 on the Development, Fluency, and Total scores. Internal consistency coefficients for the writers' scores range from .57 to .70. Coefficients were higher for both the raters' and writers' scores at higher grades. Interrater reliability coefficient averages range from .67 to .71 and thus are lower than desirable. Alternate form reliability coefficients are below acceptable standards, ranging from .39 to .52. Form B was found to be more difficult than Form A, such that the authors portray them as alternate rather than equivalent forms.

Validity. The authors describe content, concurrent, predictive, and construct validity for the WPT. They provide a rationale for the test format, writing prompts, and scoring methods, citing research and theory related to the writing process. Scores on the WPT and TOWL–2, completed by 99 students in Grades 1 through 12, were correlated to demonstrate concurrent validity, with many resulting coefficients above .40. To assess predictive validity, the WPT was administered to fourth-grade children in regular and learning disabilities classrooms. Using discriminant function analysis, the WPT scores were generally accurate in classifying children with and without learning disabilities. Factor analyses demonstrated that the Development and Fluency scales may not measure distinctive aspects of writing and thus may lack construct validity.

Critique

The WPT reflects the current emphasis on both the writing process and product. Although the test format and prompts appear appropriate, the WPT does not consistently meet acceptable standards in regard to normative procedures or reliability. Validity data are helpful but inconclusive. Additional studies to better establish reliability and validity are needed before the WPT is used on a large-scale basis for making diagnostic or classification decisions. It appears to have utility at present within a curriculum-based assessment system to monitor writing progress of individual students (S. Ward, 1998).

References

Anastasi, A., & Urbina, S. (1997). *Psychological testing* (7th ed.). New York: Macmillan.

Bain, A. M. (1988). Written expression. In K. A. Kavale, S. R. Forness, & M. Bender (Eds.), *Handbook of learning disabilities* (Vol. 2, pp. 73–88). Austin, TX: PRO-ED.

Boder, E., & Jarrico, S. (1982). *Boder Test of Reading–Spelling Patterns: A Diagnostic Screening Test for Subtypes of Reading Disability.* Orlando, FL: Psychological Corporation.

Bucy, J. E. (1998). Review of the Test of Written Language–3. In J. D. Impara & B. S. Plake (Eds.), *Thirteenth mental measurements yearbook* (pp. 1072–1074). Lincoln: Buros Institute of Mental Measurements, University of Nebraska.

California Test Bureau. (1973). *California Short-Form Test of Academic Aptitude.* Monterey, CA: Author.

Education for All Handicapped Children Act of 1975, 20 U.S.C. § 1400 *et seq.*

Hammill, D. D., Brown, V. L., Larsen, S. C., & Weiderholt, J. L. (1994). *Test of Adolescent and Adult Language–Third Edition*. Austin, TX: PRO-ED.

Hammill, D. D., & Hresko, W. P. (1994). *Comprehensive Scales of Student Abilities*. Austin, TX: PRO-ED.

Hammill, D. D., & Larsen, S. C. (1996). *Test of Written Language–Third Edition*. Austin, TX: PRO-ED.

Hansen, J. B. (1998). Review of the Test of Written Language–3. In J. D. Impara & B. S. Plake (Eds.), *Thirteenth mental measurements yearbook* (pp. 1070–1072). Lincoln: Buros Institute of Mental Measurements, University of Nebraska.

Hresko, W. P., Herron, S. R., & Peak, P. K. (1996). *Test of Early Written Language–Second Edition*. Austin, TX: PRO-ED.

Hurford, D. P. (1998). Review of the Test of Early Written Language–2. In J. D. Impara & B. S. Plake (Eds.), *Thirteenth mental measurements yearbook* (pp. 1027–1030). Lincoln: Buros Institute of Mental Measurements, University of Nebraska.

Larsen, S. C., Hammill, D. D., & Moats, L. (1999). *Test of Written Spelling–Fourth Edition*. Austin, TX: PRO-ED.

Mabry, L. (1995). Review of the Wide Range Achievement Test–3. In J. C. Conoley & J. C. Impara (Eds.), *Twelfth mental measurements yearbook* (pp. 1108–1110). Lincoln: Buros Institute of Mental Measurements, University of Nebraska.

Mather, N., & Woodcock, R. W. (1997). *Group writing tests*. Itasca, IL: Riverside.

McGhee, R., Bryant, B. R., Larsen, S. C., & Rivera, D. M. (1995). *Test of Written Expression*. Austin, TX: PRO-ED.

McGrew, K. S., Werder, J. K., & Woodcock, R. W. (1991). *WJ–R technical manual*. Allen, TX: DLM.

Perlman, C. (1998). Review of the Test of Written Expression. In J. D. Impara & B. S. Plake (Eds.), *Thirteenth mental measurements yearbook* (pp. 1068–1069). Lincoln: Buros Institute of Mental Measurements, University of Nebraska.

Psychological Corporation. (1992). *Wechsler Individual Achievement Test*. San Antonio, TX: Author.

Richards, R. A. (1998). Review of the Test of Adolescent and Adult Language–3. In J. D. Impara & B. S. Plake (Eds.), *Thirteenth mental measurements yearbook* (pp. 1019–1021). Lincoln: Buros Institute of Mental Measurements, University of Nebraska.

Salvia, J., & Ysseldyke, J. E. (1991). *Assessment* (5th ed.). Boston: Houghton Mifflin.

Taylor, S., Frackenpohl, H., White, C., Nieroroda, B., Browning, C., & Birsner, E. (1979). *EDL core vocabularies in reading, mathematics, science, and social studies*. Elmsford, NY: Arista.

Torgesen, J. K., & Bryant, B. R. (1994). *Test of Phonological Awareness*. Austin, TX: PRO-ED.

Trevisan, M. S. (1998). Review of the Test of Early Written Language–2. In J. D. Impara & B. S. Plake (Eds.), *Thirteenth mental measurements yearbook* (pp. 1030–1031). Lincoln: Buros Institute of Mental Measurements, University of Nebraska.

Ward, A. W. (1995). Review of the Wide Range Achievement Test–3. In J. C. Conoley & J. C. Impara (Eds.), *Twelfth mental measurements yearbook* (pp. 1110–1111). Lincoln: Buros Institute of Mental Measurements, University of Nebraska.

Ward, S. (1998). Review of the Writing Process Test. In J. D. Impara & B. S. Plake (Eds.), *Thirteenth mental measurements yearbook* (pp. 1161–1162). Lincoln: Buros Institute of Mental Measurements, University of Nebraska.

Warden, R., & Hutchinson, T. A. (1992). *Writing Process Test*. Itasca, IL: Riverside.

Wechsler, D. (1991). *Wechsler Intelligence Scale for Children–Third Edition*. San Antonio, TX: Psychological Corporation.

Wilkinson, G. S. (1993). *Wide Range Achievement Test–3*. San Antonio, TX: Psychological Corporation.

Woodcock, R. W., & Johnson, M. B. (1989). *Woodcock–Johnson–Revised Tests of Achievement*. Itasca, IL: Riverside.

Appendix
Principles of English Spelling

Louisa Cook Moats

Spelling Rules

1. One-syllable words ending in *f, l,* or *s,* preceded by a short vowel, usually double the final letter.

    Examples: *stuff, pill, grass, well, moss*

2. When a one-syllable word with one vowel ends in one consonant, double the final consonant before adding a suffix beginning with a vowel.

    Examples: *batter, hopping, sunned, wettest, puppy*

3. When a root word ends in a silent *e,* drop the *e* when adding a suffix beginning with a vowel. Keep the *e* before a suffix beginning with a consonant.

    Examples: *deleted, hoping, maker, famous, spicy, wasteful, extremely, excitement*

4. When a root word ends in a *y* preceded by a consonant, change the *y* to *i* before a suffix, except *–ing.* If the root word ends in a *y* preceded by a vowel, just add the suffix.

    Examples: *happiest, prettier, merriment, joyful, crying, player*

5. Use *i* before *e,* except after *c,* or when it says /a/, as in *neighbor* and *weigh.*

    Examples: *believe, piece, receive, deceive, sleigh*

Six Types of Syllables

Closed (VC). A closed syllable has only one vowel and ends in a consonant. The vowel is usually short: *com, fol, sug, trun, ject, ment.*

Silent-e (Vce). A silent-*e* syllable has one vowel followed by a consonant, followed by an *e.* The *e* is silent and makes the preceding vowel long: *vide, nize, gate, lete, mute.*

Open (CV). An open syllable ends in one vowel. The vowel is usually long: *di, re, flu, si.*

r-Controlled (Vr). An *r*-controlled syllable has a vowel followed by an *r*, which modifies the vowel sound: *der, or, par.*

Consonant-le (Cle). A consonant-*le* syllable is a final syllable in which the *e* is silent; thus, it sounds like a consonant-*l*: *sim-ple, horri-ble, un-cle.*

Double-Vowel (VV). A double-vowel syllable has two vowel letters that make one vowel sound: *pie, boat, toy, snout.*

Syllabication Rules

VC/CV. When two or more consonants stand between two vowels, divide between the two consonants, keeping blends and digraphs together: *sup / per, com / ment, en / close, diph / thong.*

V/CV. When a single consonant is surrounded by two vowels, the most common division is before the consonant, making the vowel in the first syllable long: *ro / ver, o / pen, hu / mor, ba / con.*

VC/V. If the V/CV syllable division does not make a recognizable word, divide after the consonant and give the vowel its short sound: *fab / ulous, sol / id, riv / er, gen / erate.*

/Cle. Divide before the consonant-*le*. Count back three letters from the end of the word and divide: *bu / gle, lit / tle, noo / dle, gar / gle.*

V/V. Only a few words divide between vowels: *qui / et, flu / id, po / et.*

Note: Prefixes and suffixes usually form separate syllables.

The preceding information about spelling rules, types of syllables, and syllabication rules, as well as lists of phonograms and spelling generalizations, can be found in C. Forbes's *Graded and Classified Spelling Lists for Teachers*; J. Rudd's *Word Attack Manual*; and L. Rudginsky and E. Haskell's *How to Teach Spelling*. Each of these books can be obtained from Educators Publishing Service, 75 Moulton Street, Cambridge, MA 02138-1104.

Glossary

Affix. One or more sounds or letters occurring as a bound form attached to the beginning or the end of a word, base, or phrase, which serves to produce a derivative word or inflectional form.

Coarticulation. The shaping process that naturally occurs in word pronunciation, whereby the pronunciation of one phoneme in a word exerts articulatory influence over pronunciation of adjacent phonemes.

Coherence. The quality of orderly relationships among parts of a text, and the communicative relationship between the writer and his or her audience.

Cohesion. Structures that logically relate one sentence to another within a text. Cohesive ties across sentences can be grammatical, transitional, or lexical.

Derivational Affix. A prefix or suffix that is added to a base word form to modify its meaning or to change its part of speech. More than one derivational affix may be added to a single base form.

Dysgraphia. A disorder in visual–motor integration, characterized by an inability to copy as well as to write from memory.

Grapheme. A written alphabet letter, of which there are 26 in the English language.

Graphemic Unit. Any single alphabet letter or group of letters that represents a single phoneme. For example, graphemic units *i, k,* and *ck* each can represent the /k/ sound, depending upon its location within a given word.

Inflectional Suffix. A suffix that does not change the part of speech of the base form to which it is attached. Only one inflectional suffix may be added to the base word at a time. These suffixes serve to change the person or the tense of a verb, to signify plural or possessive forms, and to form comparative and superlative word forms.

Lexical. 1. Of or relating to words, or the vocabulary of the language. 2. The meaning of the base word in derived or inflected forms, such as *plays, played, playing*.

Morpheme. A meaningful linguistic unit, whether in a free form such as *pin*, or a bound form such as the *s* in *pins*. A linguistic part containing no smaller meaningful parts.

Morphology. The system of word formation in a language; the study of word formation patterns.

Orthographic Marker. A graphemic unit of one or more alphabet letters whose function is to indicate pronunciation of a preceding grapheme, such as the silent *e* in *race*, or to preserve visual similarities in the spellings of related word forms, such as *g* in *sign* and *signal*. Orthographic markers by definition always are silent.

Orthographics. 1. The art of writing words, with proper letters according to standard usage. 2. A part of language study that deals with letters and spelling.

Phoneme. A speech sound in a language, which is recognized by speakers as changing meaning of contrasting pairs of words, such as *bin–pin*.

Phonetics. The study and systematic classification of the sounds made in spoken utterances; the way in which the sound is articulated.

Phonics. The science of sound; the method of teaching beginners to read and to pronounce words by learning the phonetic value of letters, letter groups, and especially syllables.

Phonological Rules. Those rules that govern the production of sounds in a language.

Reliability. A measure of the degree to which a test consistently measures what it purports to measure; also, the degree to which a test is free from random measurement error.

Semantics. The study of word meanings.

Syllable. A unit of language that is next bigger than a speech sound and consists of one or more vowel sounds alone, or one or more consonant sounds preceding or following the vowel sound.

Syntax. The way in which words are put together to form phrases and sentences.

Validity. The degree to which a test measures what its author or authors claim it measures.

Index

About the Authors

Ann M. Bain, EdD, has been working with children with learning disabilities for over 30 years. She received her EdD in Human Communication and Its Disorders from Johns Hopkins University in 1982 and has been a fellow of the Academy of Orton-Gillingham Practitioners and Educators since 1996. She is the recipient of the Dr. Robert M. N. Crosby Award as well as the Distinguished Alumna Award from Albertus Magnus College. She is the author of several articles, chapters, and workbooks. She also has given presentations across the country, specializing in written language disorders and other learning disabilities. She has taught many graduate as well as undergraduate courses in special education at Loyola College and Johns Hopkins University. Dr. Bain is on the faculty in the Graduate Education Division at Goucher College. She is a diagnostic prescriptive specialist at Sheppard Pratt Health System in Baltimore, Maryland, where she evaluates children's learning needs and trains and supervises teachers.

Louisa Cook Moats holds an EdD from the Harvard University Graduate School of Education. She is currently the Washington, DC, site director for a 5-year study of early reading instruction conducted in the Houston and Washington, DC, public schools funded by the National Institute of Child Health and Human Development under the leadership of Dr. Barbara Foorman (HD 33095). She holds the position of clinical associate professor of pediatrics at the University of Texas Health Sciences Center in Houston. Dr. Moats has been a teacher, psychologist, consultant, author, and researcher specializing in reading, writing, and learning disorders. A recognized expert in her field, she lectures and teaches widely across the United States and abroad, and has published several books on spelling, language, and dyslexia. She is coauthor of the *Test of Written Spelling–Fourth Edition* (PRO-ED), the *Scholastic Spelling Program,* and the new spelling and writing components of *Language!* (Sopris West).

Laura Lyons Bailet received her PhD in communicative disorders from Northwestern University, with a specialization in learning disabilities. She has worked with individuals with learning disorders for 20 years, as both a teacher and a licensed school psychologist. She currently directs the Neurocognitive Testing Program within the Neurology division of the Nemours Children's Clinic in Jacksonville, Florida, which focuses on psychoeducational assessment of children with learning problems. She has published journal articles and book chapters on spelling disabilities and on cognitive

263

deficits associated with childhood epilepsy. Her current interests include dyslexia, autism–spectrum disorders, cognitive and academic achievement problems associated with pediatric medical conditions, and early intervention for preschoolers with developmental delays. She presents frequently on these topics at local and regional conferences.